How to Cook
for Crohn's and Colitis

How to Cook for Crohn's and Colitis

More Than 200 Healthy, Delicious Recipes the Whole Family Will Love

Brenda Roscher

CUMBERLAND HOUSE
AN IMPRINT OF SOURCEBOOKS, INC.®

PUBLISHED BY CUMBERLAND HOUSE PUBLISHING, AN IMPRINT OF SOURCEBOOKS, INC.
PO Box 4410
Naperville, Il 60567-4410

Cover design: JulesRulesDesign
Text design: Lisa Taylor

Library of Congress Cataloging-in-Publication Data

Roscher, Brenda, 1959–
  How to cook for Crohn's and colitis : more than 200 healthy, delicious recipes the whole family will love / Brenda Roscher.
      p. cm.
  Includes bibligraphical references and index.
1. Crohn's disease—Diet therapy—Recipes. 2. Colitis—Diet therapy—Recipes. I. Title.

  RC862.E52R67 2007
  616.3'440654—dc22

                                                                                    2007028669

Printed in the United States of America
DR 10 9 8 7 6

For all those diagnosed with inflammatory bowel disease and their families. I hope that the information and recipes found here allow you to enjoy food again.

Contents

Foreword

As a physician, it has always been my privilege to be inspired by my patients' responses to their illnesses. Since I specialize in treating patients with Crohn's disease and ulcerative colitis, I am given more than ample opportunity to witness remarkable feats of recovery and renewal in between periods of catastrophic relapses.

I think it is impossible not to be inspired by Brenda Roscher's story of an unexpected diagnosis of severe Crohn's disease, which nearly ended her life. Brenda's story is ultimately a love story in that her love of food and the joy that she derived from it could not be overcome by her severe physical illness. Once Brenda was able to recover, she courageously faced the new reality of her plumbing and learned how to love food again. Like a mountain climber who has taken a bad tumble, a skier who has broken a leg, or a surfer who has encountered a shark, she jumped right back into the game, and all of us get to benefit from her bravery.

The recipes in this cookbook are well thought out and nutritious and would, I think, do proud the dinner table of anyone who loves food, whether they have Crohn's disease and ulcerative colitis or not. So I urge you to read and get cooking—bon appétit!

—James F. Marion, MD
Assistant Clinical Professor of Medicine
Mount Sinai School of Medicine

Introduction: My Story

I was diagnosed with Crohn's disease in December 2001. My symptoms, though, had begun two years earlier. In the fall of 1999, I had diarrhea and pain in my abdomen every day for a month. I felt tired all the time. I thought it was the flu or that I had a bug that I just couldn't shake. I saw a doctor. He poked around my belly and then told me it was probably gall bladder disease (common for women my age). Thanks so much! He suggested a bland diet that included cutting down on fats. The pain, however, continued to come and go, sometimes being unbearable. The diarrhea didn't stop, and the gas—oh my God! I kept wondering when I was going to pass those gall stones!

There was a heaviness in my lower abdomen, and my abdominal pain worsened, especially when trying to poo, which was most of the time. I returned to my regular doctor, and after an exam and blood work, she sent me off to have both external and internal ultrasounds. They found nothing other than I had a lot of gas. News flash! I just wasn't getting any answers. For about a year and a half I went on living with the symptoms. I lost twenty-five pounds.

In September 2001, my husband Dan and I moved to Myrtle Beach from Charleston, SC. Setting up a new household is stressful. Finding your way around a new city is stressful. Looking for a new job is stressful. And the move was particularly stressful for me because I was moving away from my daughters. Though they were adults (eighteen and twenty years old), they were still my babies.

On Christmas Day Dan and I invited a friend over to share turkey with all the trimmings. I made it through preparing the feast, even ate a little, and then excused myself to lie down. I couldn't do any more because of the pain. I thought, *Maybe this is it, maybe I'm finally going to pass those gall stones, or maybe it's appendicitis, or maybe I'm going to poop myself to death!*

For the next couple of days, it was all I could do to get out of bed to get to the bathroom because the pain was so intense. Then it happened. A pain shot through me like someone had stabbed me the gut and was twisting the blade. I gasped for breath. Dan rushed me to the hospital. I woke up in the ICU with a catheter; a tube down my nose into my stomach; IVs in my legs, arms, and belly; my abdomen distended and terribly painful. The doctor told me I had nearly died of a disease I had never heard of: Crohn's.

Five days later I was released from the hospital with prescriptions for antibiotics, steroids, painkillers, and acid reducers. The only information on Crohn's disease I received before leaving the hospital was that Crohn's is believed to be an autoimmune disease that affects the digestive tract. Surgery is often performed—sometimes repeatedly—and there is no cure.

When I returned home, I had a lot of questions. What exactly *is* Crohn's? What are the symptoms? What causes it? Is there anything I can do to control it? And most immediately, what can I eat? What can't I eat? That's when my research began.

1. Crohn's Disease and Ulcerative Colitis

Crohn's disease is named for Burrill Bernard Crohn after he and others described it in a published article in 1932. It is also referred to as ileitis. Crohn's disease is an inflammation of the digestive tract. It occurs most frequently in the small intestine, although it can appear anywhere from the mouth to the anus. Crohn's and its sister disease, ulcerative colitis, fall under the umbrella of inflammatory bowel disease (IBD). Crohn's and colitis share similar symptoms, but colitis differs in that it usually affects only the colon and rectum. IBD is a chronic disease and should not be confused with IBS (irritable bowel syndrome), which has some similar symptoms. IBS does not have the serious complications of IBD, nor is it medically treated the same way. During an attack of IBD—or "flare-up," as it is commonly called—any of the following symptoms can occur:

Symptoms of IBD
- diarrhea
- low-grade fever
- fatigue
- loss of appetite
- abdominal cramping and pain
- weight loss
- flatulence (gas)
- blood in the stool
- headaches
- vomiting

Complications of IBD
- malabsorption (nutrients are poorly absorbed)
- steatorrhea (excess fat not absorbed, creating floating stool)
- peritonitis (intestinal wall leaks)
- strictures (partial obstruction of the bowel)

- fistulas and abscesses (abnormal passages that lead from one loop to another or even to other organs)
- iron-deficiency anemia
- malnutrition

Theories of What Causes Crohn's and Colitis
- **Genetic Factors**: Twenty percent of patients have a close family member with the disease. It is also more prevalent in those of European and Jewish descent.
- **Virus** or bacterium that causes the immune system to produce antibodies that attack the digestive tract.
- **Environmental Factors**: The disease is found more frequently in industrialized nations and in those whose diet consists of high-fat and refined foods.

Possible Contributing Factors
- smoking
- oral contraceptive use
- MMR vaccine (Measles-Mumps-Rubella)
- antibiotic use
- zinc deficiency

Crohn's and Colitis by the Numbers
An estimated 1.4 million Americans have Crohn's or colitis with 30,000 new cases diagnosed each year. It is most commonly diagnosed in people between the ages of 15–35. It occurs about equally between men and women. Conditions associated with IBD are arthritis, migraines, kidney stones, and osteoporosis, among others. Crohn's and colitis patients also have a higher risk of developing colon cancer. IBD has increased rapidly since the 1950s, and this could be because of environmental factors or better diagnosis of the disease.

Diagnosis
After a complete physical and blood tests, your doctor will probably order a barium x-ray and a colonoscopy. A barium x-ray consists of drinking liquid barium on an empty stomach prior to a series of x-rays. In a colonoscopy, a flexible tube with a scope on the end is inserted in your rectum so that the entire colon can be examined for inflammation and obstructions.

Treatments
Research is ongoing for new drugs to better treat the symptoms of Crohn's and colitis.

Currently, the most common treatments are:

- **Immunosuppressives**: Azathioprine (Imuran), 6-mercaptopurine (6-mp), and Infliximab (Remicade) suppress the immune system and reduce inflammation.
- **Antibiotics**: Metronidazole (Flagyl) and Ciprofloxacin (Cipro) are effective in treating abscesses and fistulas in Crohn's but have little affect on colitis.
- **Anti-inflammatories**: Sulfasalazine (5-ASA) and Corticosteroids, as the name suggests, reduce inflammation in the intestines.

These treatments can cause a host of side effects ranging from mild to severe. Yet these drugs can get you closer to "normal." Trust in your doctor but don't be afraid to ask questions.

Other Medications and Supplements Used to Reduce Symptoms

Please talk to your doctor before taking any over-the-counter drug. This is not a disclaimer—this is serious, especially during flare-ups!

- **Nicotine patches**: Although smoking is thought to be a contributor to Crohn's (especially in women), nicotine patches have been used to temporarily relieve the symptoms of colitis.
- **Antidiarrheal drugs (Imodium)**: Slow down muscle activity, and fiber (Metamucil) bulks up stool.
- **Laxatives**: In cases of constipation.
- **Acetaminophen (Tylenol)**: For pain relief.
- **H-2 blockers (Pepcid, Tagamet, Zantac)**: Acid reducers.
- **Multivitamins and/or iron supplements**: For deficiencies caused by diarrhea and inadequate nutrient intake and in cases of iron-deficiency anemia.

Surgery

When other treatments fail, surgery may be recommended. With Crohn's, removing the portion the gastro-intestinal tract that is damaged can result in remission of the disease, but it may only be temporary. The disease may recur and further surgery may be necessary. With colitis, the disease can be "cured" by removal of the entire colon and rectum.

Nutritional Treatments

- **Elemental Diet**: A liquid diet in which all essential nutrients (proteins, carbohydrates, fats) are provided in predigested form.
- **Total Parenteral Nutrition (TPN)**: For seriously ill patients, a liquid diet fed intravenously.

Stress and Depression

Stress and depression do not cause IBD, but they can exacerbate symptoms. They also can be an effect of the limitation the disease can impose on the quality of one's life. Constantly needing bathroom facilities nearby, embarrassment, fatigue, reduced appetite, abdominal pain, etc., can make people with IBD feel both physically and emotionally homebound and isolated.

Here are some ideas to consider to manage stress and depression:

Relaxation Techniques
- deep breathing
- yoga
- meditation
- Tai Chi
- listening to music
- reading

Inform Yourself and Talk with Others

The more you know about your disease, the more you will feel in control of your life. Seek support from family, friends, and fellow IBD sufferers. Contact the CCFA (Crohn's and Colitis Foundation of America) for a chapter near you. Also, Web site resources are listed on page 218.

Lifestyle
- Do you need to work fifty hours a week? Could you get by on forty hours?
- Frequently eating on the run? Make time to prepare a meal and sit down to eat.
- Feel as though you're spread too thin with obligations to others? Learn to say no.
- Set aside thirty minutes every day to do something you love. For me it's cooking, playing guitar, and solving crossword puzzles.
- Feel like you don't have time to exercise? Take a walk after dinner or toss a ball around with the kids in the backyard. Even simple, regular exercise can help.

Diet and Nutrition

Adequate nutrition is of serious concern for people with Crohn's and colitis, especially during flare-ups. When suffering from abdominal pain, chronic diarrhea, and lack of appetite, it can be a challenge to consume the nutrients your body needs. Sometimes iron-deficiency anemia and even malnutrition can occur.

There is no evidence that a particular food or group of foods causes Crohn's and colitis, yet certain foods—or the way they are prepared—can aggravate symptoms. Keeping a food diary for a few weeks is a good way to track not only what you have consumed but also how your body reacts. Keep in mind that the total digestive process can take up to forty-eight hours, beginning in the stomach within thirty minutes to two hours of ingestion and ending twelve to forty-eight hours later with elimination. Because of the time frame involved in digestion, you may not have an immediate reaction as in the case of a severe food allergy. Your body may be reacting today from that heavenly fettuccini alfredo you had last night at Luigi's.

Lactose Intolerance

Lactose intolerance occurs when the body doesn't produce enough of the enzyme lactase to break down lactose, the sugar found in dairy products. The most common symptoms of lactose intolerance are gas, bloating, abdominal pain, and diarrhea. The symptoms usually begin thirty minutes to two hours after consuming food or drink containing lactose. Not all persons with IBD are also lactose intolerant, but many are. Keeping a food diary can help you ascertain if you are. Try eliminating dairy products for several days, and then reintroduce them gradually, noting any symptoms. The only problem with this is that many processed products, even if they don't contain whole milk, may contain hidden dairy in the form of dried milk solids or whey, for example.

Talk to your doctor. If you think you might be lactose intolerant, (s)he can diagnose it with one or more of the following tests:

- Lactose intolerance test
- Hydrogen breath test
- Stool acidity test

If you find that you are indeed lactose intolerant, there are steps you can take to ensure you are getting enough calcium in your diet.

Calcium-Rich and Low-Lactose Foods

- **Yogurt:** Contains active bacteria that produce lactase to digest lactose.
- **Aged Cheeses:** The aging process includes bacteria that lowers lactose. Sharp Cheddar, Swiss, and Parmesan are good choices.
- **Whole Milk Substitutes:** Lactose-free milk, soy milk, and rice milk are readily available at supermarkets. They tend to be a bit sweeter than whole milk.
- **Enzyme Products:** Lactase drops can be added to milk, and lactase tablets can be taken with meals containing lactose.
- **Non-Dairy Calcium-Rich Foods:** Sardines, salmon, green leafy vegetables, beans, and soybean products are good sources of calcium.

Keep in mind that low fat does not equal low lactose. In fact, quite the opposite can be true.

Protein

Every cell in the body requires protein for growth and repair. It is needed to produce antibodies, enzymes, and some hormones. Proteins are broken down into two groups:

- **Complete**: containing all essential amino acids, and
- **Incomplete**: containing some essential amino acids. There are twenty amino acids the body requires to form protein. Of these, eleven are produced within the body, and nine (essential) must come from diet. Combining two incomplete proteins—beans and rice, for example—will create a complete protein.

Good Sources of Complete Protein

- lean meats
- lean chicken
- fresh fish
- canned tuna
- dairy products
- eggs
- soy products

Good Sources of Incomplete Protein

- beans
- nut butters
- rice
- pasta

Carbohydrates

Carbohydrates supply the body with energy in the form of glucose and are, for the most part, derived from plants. The major exception to this is lactose in milk. Carbohydrates are broken down into two groups: simple and complex.

Simple carbohydrates are digested quickly and occur naturally in berries, some vegetables, and honey, or in the form of processed table sugar and lactose from dairy products. Complex carbohydrates take a little longer to digest and are composed of starches and fiber found in vegetables and grains.

Fiber

Fiber is important to healthy digestion and colon function. Dietary fiber comes in two forms: soluble and insoluble. Soluble fiber dissolves in water and can be found in fruits, beans, legumes, oat bran, etc. Insoluble fiber does not dissolve in water and passes through the digestive tract essentially unchanged. It can be found in vegetables, nuts, wheat bran, brown rice, and the skin of fruits.

Increasing the fiber content in the diet may reduce the risk of colon cancer, yet for people with IBD, there are a few things to consider.

- Try adding more fiber to your diet gradually. A sudden increase in fiber consumption can produce gas, bloating, and constipation.
- Try oatmeal, potato, sourdough, or French breads. Wheat bran and other whole grains are insoluble fibers and may be rough on the digestive tract, especially during a flare-up. Popcorn is also an insoluble fiber and can be difficult to digest.
- Whole nuts can be difficult to digest. Nut butters may be better tolerated.
- Canned beans contain less indigestible sugars than dried beans and, therefore, are less gas producing.
- Some vegetables—especially those in the cabbage family, such as broccoli and cauliflower—and some raw fruits, such as apples, are known for causing gas. Talk to your doctor about taking Beano or an acid reducer before consuming them.

Dietary Fats

Fats are needed for many chemical activities including regulating body temperature, organ protection, and hormone production. Fats also make foods more flavorful and satisfying. Dietary fats are broken down into three groups: saturated, monounsaturated, and polyunsaturated.

Most saturated fats (meats, butter, coconut and palm oils) are solid at room temperature or when chilled—with the exception of tropical oils. They are considered to be the main constituent of high cholesterol.

Monounsaturated fats (canola, olive, and sesame seed oils) are liquid at room temperature and solidify under refrigeration. These fats lower cholesterol.

Polyunsaturated fats are rich in Omega 6 fatty acids (corn, safflower, and sunflower oils) and Omega 3 fatty acids (fish, flaxseed, and canola oils) and are almost always liquid whether at room temperature or chilled. The exception to this is when the oil undergoes hydrogenation (a process by which hydrogen atoms are added) and becomes a solid such as margarine or vegetable shortening. Hydrogenated oils are referred to as trans fats and behave more like saturated fats.

Currently, a myriad of benefits are being touted for Omega 3 fatty acids in particular, including lowering cholesterol, reducing inflammation in arthritis, and even reducing some symptoms of Crohn's.

I think the best thing to come out of the low-carb craze is the availability of the butter/canola oil blend. It delivers the wonderful taste of butter with the benefit of less saturated fat. It can be used in cooking and baking or as a spread just like regular butter.

Fluids

Diarrhea can cause a rapid loss of water in the body. It's important to replace lost fluids so you don't become dehydrated. Water, teas, and clear fruit juices are the best choices. Citrus juices can be irritating to the digestive tract. Filtered or spring water may be beneficial if you are uncertain of the purity of your tap water. Caffeine can stimulate the intestines which, in turn, can make diarrhea worse. If you love your coffee, switch to decaffeinated. At the very least, switch to a reduced-caffeine coffee and have one cup instead of two or three. Carbonated drinks are not a good option because they are gas producing and most contain caffeine.

Alcohol

Alcohol can stimulate the intestines; therefore, during a flare-up you might want to limit your consumption. I won't make a blanket statement and say eliminate all alcoholic beverages, but I will say the following of beer, liquor, and wine. Beer causes bloating. Distilled liquor has the highest alcohol content of the three and is usually served with a mixer such as soda. Wine, on the upside, is rich in antioxidants, which offer protection from heart disease and cancer. Wine also increases "good" cholesterol. On the downside, most wines contain sulfites which can trigger nausea and diarrhea. Personally, I enjoy wine and I'm going to continue to enjoy wine. The decision of whether to consume alcohol is entirely up to you.

Teas

Black, green, and white teas have about half the caffeine of coffee. They are high in antioxidants, which protect against heart disease and cancer. Green tea also contains high levels of vitamin K, which is necessary for proper blood clotting. Herbal teas are caffeine-free, and some are known for the calming effect on the digestive tract. Chamomile is a digestive and mild sedative. Lemon balm is calming and relieves gas. Peppermint is a digestive and relieves gas. (Please note that peppermint tea should not be consumed by someone with hiatal hernia). Fennel is also a digestive and reduces gas.

Herbs and Spices

Besides adding great flavor to foods, herbs have been used for centuries for their medicinal properties. Garlic, for example, is a digestive that inhibits the growth of harmful bacteria in the intestines and supports the growth of good bacteria. The following are some common herbs and spices that aid digestion.

- basil
- bay leaf
- black pepper

- cinnamon
- coriander
- cumin
- dill
- ginger
- oregano
- parsley
- rosemary
- sage
- thyme

Probiotics

Probiotics are living "friendly" bacteria that help provide a balance of intestinal flora. The most common food that contains probiotics is yogurt. When shopping for yogurt, look for a label that reads "live active cultures." There are many benefits of this food:
- It is an easily digested protein.
- It is a great source of calcium.
- It reduces diarrhea, including diarrhea associated with antibiotic use.
- It is usually well tolerated even by those who are lactose intolerant.

Preservatives and Additives

Preservatives and additives are used in foods to enhance flavor, improve texture, extend shelf life and make them more visually appealing. Many have no adverse effects on our health and, in fact, make foods safer for our consumption. However, some may have adverse effects, especially for IBD's. Some examples:
- **Carrageenan:** Stabilizer used in many dairy products. It also has been used to induce colitis in guinea pigs.
- **Guar Gum:** Thickening agent that can cause excess gas, nausea, and abdominal cramps.
- **Gum Arabic:** Stabilizer that can cause excess gas.
- **Olestra:** Fat substitute that can cause diarrhea and abdominal cramping.
- **Sorbitol:** Sugar substitute that can cause excess gas and diarrhea.
- **Sulfites:** Preservative that can cause diarrhea and nausea.

I'm not implying that any particular preservative or additive is a cause of IBD, only that some *could* aggravate symptoms of IBD. Become an avid label reader. By reading food labels you become keenly aware of the contents of the prepackaged foods you are eating. (Please see Further Reading on page 218 for more information concerning preservatives and additives.)

In Conclusion - Dietary Suggestions
Eating Habits
- Having 5–6 smaller meals rather than 3 large ones may be beneficial during a flare-up.
- Chewing gum, using a straw for drinks, and gulping food can cause gas and bloating from excess air intake.
- Slow down and chew food well, just like your mom told you to.

Fluids
- Drink 8–10 glasses of fluids every day to avoid dehydration.
- Water is best. Filtered or spring water may be beneficial.
- Teas and clear fruit juices are also good choices.
- Reduce consumption of caffeinated and carbonated beverages.

Supplements
- Talk to your doctor about taking a multivitamin. Also ask about a fish oil or flaxseed oil supplement as they are rich in Omega 3 fatty acids known for their anti-inflammatory properties.

Lactose Intolerance
- Yogurt contains "friendly" bacteria that help provide a balance of intestinal flora and is usually well tolerated by those who are lactose intolerant.
- Aged cheeses such as Cheddar, Swiss and Parmesan are low lactose.
- Experiment with lactose-free, soy, and rice milks and/or enzyme products.
- Generally, the lower the fat in dairy products, the higher the lactose content.

Dietary Fats
- Think good fats—monounsaturated fats like canola, olive, and sesame oils and Omega-3 rich polyunsaturated fats like fish, flaxseed, and canola oils.
- Reduce saturated fats—butter, tropical oils, and hydrogenated fats (trans fats), such as margarine and shortening. Many processed foods contain these fats. Check the ingredient list on packages of potato and corn chips, crackers, cookies, and other snack and convenience foods.
- Substitute a butter/canola oil blend for whole butter. It works and tastes the same and contains less saturated fat.
- Substitute a salad dressing such as Miracle Whip or a low-fat mayonnaise for regular mayonnaise.
- Whole nuts can be difficult to digest. Try natural, creamy-style nut butters (no hy-

drogenated oils). Although nut butters are relatively high in fat, they are low in saturated fat.

- Chocolate is high in fat. If you are a die-hard fan of chocolate, use cocoa or carob powder in baking. Both have little to no fat, depending on the brand you choose.

Carbohydrates

- Raw fruits, such as apples, and vegetables, especially those in the cabbage family including broccoli and cauliflower, can cause gas. Talk to your doctor about taking Beano or an acid reducer before consuming them.
- Beans are a good source of protein and soluble fiber and are low in fat. They also can produce gas. Canned beans, rinsed well and drained, are a better choice than dried beans because some of the gas producing sugars (oligosaccharides) are removed during processing.
- Oatmeal, potato, sourdough, and French breads are examples of soluble fiber and are easier to digest than whole wheat or multi-grain breads, which are insoluble fiber. This doesn't mean total elimination of whole grains from the diet, but during a flare-up breads made from white flour may be better tolerated.
- Popcorn is also an insoluble fiber and difficult to digest.
- When adding more fiber to your diet, do so gradually. A sudden increase can produce gas, bloating, and constipation.

Protein

- Lean meats, poultry, fish, canned tuna in water, eggs, and dairy products are all good sources of complete protein, which the body needs for growth and repair.
- Beans, nut butters, rice, and pasta are good sources of incomplete protein.
- Sauté, poach, broil, and roast meats.
- Limit consumption of deep-fat fried foods.
- Processed meats such as salami, bologna, and sausage are high in fat and in preservatives and/or additives.
- Make your own sausage at home using lean pork, chicken, or turkey.

Before You Begin

Some helpful notes about the recipes:

- With the exception of mushrooms, all vegetables should be washed before preparing, including lettuce greens and fresh herbs.
- Potatoes, carrots, and onions are peeled of their skin unless otherwise noted.
- Bell peppers are seeded.
- One medium clove of garlic equals ½ teaspoon minced garlic.

- Butter, unless otherwise noted, is a butter/canola oil blend.
- Beef and chicken broths are low sodium.
- "Trimmed" meats means trimmed of most visible fat.
- Hamburger is at least 93 percent lean.
- "Picked over" in the crab meat recipes means to gently feel the meat for any stray pieces of shell.
- Eggs are omega-3-rich large eggs.
- Flour is all-purpose white flour unless otherwise noted.
- Sugar, unless otherwise noted, is granulated.
- Most recipes contain substitution suggestions for those who are lactose intolerant.
- Most recipes are designed to be low in fat, especially saturated fat.
- In recipes that call for Miracle Whip, other salad dressings or low-fat mayonnaise may be substituted.

Layered Pinto and Black Bean Dip

Serve this favorite party dip with homemade Pita Chips or Tortilla Chips (pg. 26).

1	16-oz. can fat-free refried pinto beans
1	15-oz. can black beans, rinsed and drained
¼	teaspoon chili powder
¼	teaspoon cumin
1	cup salsa, homemade or bottled
1	cup shredded 2% sharp Cheddar cheese
1	cup Velvety Guacamole (pg. 28)
	Lite sour cream or plain yogurt (optional)
	Sliced scallions (optional)
	Chopped fresh cilantro (optional)

◉ Preheat oven to 350°F. Spread refried beans in the bottom of a glass pie plate or shallow casserole dish. Top with black beans. Sprinkle with chili powder and cumin. Spoon salsa on top of seasonings and sprinkle with Cheddar.

◉ Bake for 15–20 minutes, until Cheddar has melted. Remove from oven and spread guacamole on top of Cheddar. Garnish with sour cream, scallions, and cilantro, if desired.

Note: For a lower-lactose dip, substitute full-fat sharp Cheddar cheese for the 2% variety, and opt for plain yogurt in place of the lite sour cream.

Makes 8–10 servings, about ¼ cup each

Pita Chips

4	pita breads, split horizontally
2	tablespoons butter/canola oil blend or olive oil
$\frac{1}{2}$	teaspoon garlic powder
$\frac{1}{4}$	teaspoon salt
$\frac{1}{4}$	teaspoon black pepper

- Preheat oven to 400°F. Spread pita halves with butter or drizzle with olive oil. Cut each half into 6 wedges.

- Coat a baking sheet with vegetable spray and arrange wedges on sheet in a single layer. Sprinkle wedges with garlic powder, salt, and pepper. Bake for 8–10 minutes, until crisp.

Variation
Tortilla Chips: Substitute 8 (7- to 8-inch) flour tortillas for the pita halves and chili powder for the garlic powder. Proceed as directed.

Makes 48 chips

Fresh Tomato Salsa

For a refreshing twist, try one of the variations listed below. The addition of naturally sweet fruit takes the salsa to a whole new level.

6	medium Roma tomatoes, diced
1	4-oz. can diced green chiles, drained
1	cup diced onion (about 1 medium onion)
1	tablespoon chopped fresh cilantro
1	tablespoon fresh lime juice
1	teaspoon lime zest (grated rind)
½	teaspoon salt
¼	teaspoon cumin

◉ Combine all ingredients in a medium-sized bowl and stir well to combine. Cover and chill at least 2 hours before serving.

Variations
Blueberry Salsa: Add 1 cup fresh or frozen blueberries.
Mango Salsa: Add 1 ripe mango, peeled and diced.
Peach Salsa: Add 2 ripe peaches, pitted, peeled, and diced.

Makes about 3 cups

Velvety Guacamole

Although avocados are high in fat, they consist mainly of monounsaturated fats and have no cholesterol.

2	ripe Hass avocados, pitted*
2	tablespoons fresh lime or lemon juice
2	medium Roma tomatoes, diced
¼	cup diced onion (about ½ small onion)
2	tablespoons chopped fresh cilantro
1	teaspoon minced garlic (about 2 medium cloves)
2	tablespoons diced green chiles (optional)
¼	teaspoon cumin
¼	teaspoon salt

◉ Scoop out avocado halves into a bowl. Add lime juice and mash the avocados. Add remaining ingredients and stir well to combine. Serve immediately.

Note: Avocados are ripe when they yield to gentle pressure.

Makes about 2 cups

Hummus with Roasted Red Peppers

1	15-oz. can garbanzo beans, rinsed and drained
1	teaspoon minced garlic (about 2 medium cloves)
1	7-oz. jar roasted red peppers, drained and chopped
¼	cup tahini (sesame butter)
2	tablespoons fresh lemon juice
2	tablespoons olive oil
½	teaspoon salt
¼	teaspoon cumin
¼	teaspoon coriander
⅛	teaspoon cayenne (optional)

◉ Place beans in a food processor or blender and process until smooth. Add remaining ingredients and process until combined well.

◉ Cover and chill for at least 1 hour. Serve with Pita Chips (pg. 26).

Variations
Black Bean Hummus: Substitute black beans for the garbanzos.
Great Northern Hummus: Substitute Great Northern beans for the garbanzos.
Hummus with Sun-dried Tomatoes: Substitute half of a 7-oz. jar of sun-dried tomatoes in oil (drained and chopped) for the roasted red peppers.

Makes about 2 cups

Roasted Garlic

Garlic has been used by herbalists for centuries as a digestive and to fight or prevent infections. When roasted, garlic becomes soft, mellow, and sweet.

5	large heads garlic
2	tablespoons olive oil
¼	teaspoon salt
¼	teaspoon black pepper

◉ Heat oven to 375°F. Remove the loose, papery skin from garlic heads. Cut top off of garlic heads (about ¼-inch), leaving the bulb intact. Place garlic in a baking dish cut-side up. Drizzle with olive oil and sprinkle with salt and pepper. Cover with aluminum foil. Bake for about 1 hour.

◉ Remove from oven and remove aluminum foil. When cool enough to handle, squeeze the soft garlic out of each clove into a small serving dish or bowl. Serve with a warm, crusty loaf of bread.

Makes about 1 cup

Spinach, Swiss, and Artichoke Dip

1	bunch loose leaf spinach or 1 10-oz. bag baby spinach, chopped
1	14-oz. can artichoke hearts, drained and chopped
½	cup diced onion (about 1 small onion)
½	cup Miracle Whip
1	cup shredded Swiss cheese
½	cup lite sour cream or plain yogurt
¼	teaspoon salt
¼	teaspoon black pepper

◉ Preheat oven to 350°F. Combine all ingredients in a mixing bowl. Coat a 1½-quart casserole dish with vegetable spray. Spoon dip into casserole evenly. Bake for 20–25 minutes, until bubbly.

◉ Serve with Pita Chips (pg. 26) or assorted crackers.

Variation
Spinach, Parmesan, and Artichoke Dip: Substitute ½ cup grated Parmesan cheese for the Swiss.

Makes about 3 cups

Chilled Crab Dip

To make this dip lower lactose, substitute full-fat sharp Cheddar for the 2%, omit Neufchâtel cheese, and increase Miracle Whip to ½ cup.

1	16-oz. container lump or claw (or combination) crabmeat, picked over
1	cup 2% sharp Cheddar cheese, shredded
4	oz. Neufchâtel cheese (or other reduced-fat cream cheese), softened
⅓	cup Miracle Whip
1	tablespoon fresh lemon juice
1	teaspoon lemon zest (grated rind)
1	tablespoon Worcestershire sauce
1	teaspoon Old Bay seasoning
½	teaspoon garlic powder
½	teaspoon hot pepper sauce, such as Texas Pete or Tabasco (optional)

◉ Combine all ingredients in a medium bowl and mix well. This is most efficiently done with your hands. Cover and chill at least 1 hour. Serve with assorted crackers.

Variation
Chilled Salmon Dip: Substitute 2 cups cooked salmon for the crabmeat.

Makes about 3½ cups

Stuffed Mushrooms—Three Ways

Plain bread crumbs are readily available at your local grocery store, but check the ingredients, especially if you are lactose intolerant. Many contain ingredients such as hydrogenated oil and milk products, including whey. An alternative is to make your own and it's very simple. Heat oven to 300°F. Cube bread slices and arrange in a single layer on an ungreased baking sheet. Bake about 12–15 minutes, until dry and crispy. Let cool. Place in a plastic ziplock bag and crush using a rolling pin or mallet.

	Stuffing of choice from below
8	oz. fresh white mushrooms or baby bellas (cremini mushrooms)
1	tablespoon olive oil

◉ Heat oven to 375°F. Prepare stuffing of choice by combing stuffing ingredients in a bowl. Coat a baking sheet with vegetable spray. Brush any dirt from mushrooms with paper towel—do not wash as this will make mushrooms rubbery. Remove stems from mushrooms. Spoon stuffing into mushroom caps and place on baking sheet stuffing side up. Drizzle with olive oil.

◉ Bake for 10–15 minutes until mushrooms are soft and stuffing is heated through.

Crab Stuffing
1	8-oz. container lump or claw crabmeat, picked over
¼	cup plain bread crumbs
¼	cup grated Parmesan cheese
¼	teaspoon Old Bay seasoning
⅛	teaspoon black pepper

Sausage Stuffing
8	oz. Sweet Italian Sausage (pg. 117), cooked and drained
¼	cup plain bread crumbs
¼	cup grated Parmesan cheese
½	teaspoon minced garlic (about 1 medium clove)

Spinach Stuffing
1	10-oz. package frozen chopped spinach, thawed and squeezed dry
½	cup packaged or Seasoned Croutons (pg. 57), crushed
1	egg white
½	teaspoon minced garlic (about 1 medium clove)

Makes about 12–16 appetizers

Crostini—Three Ways

For lower lactose crostini, substitute full-fat sharp Cheddar for the mozzarella and grated Parmesan cheese for the feta.

8   (1-inch) slices French or rustic bread, preferably sliced at an angle

1   tablespoon butter/canola oil blend or olive oil

2   teaspoons minced garlic (about 4 medium cloves)

Topping of choice from below

◉ Set oven to broil. Place bread slices on baking sheet. Spread slices with butter or drizzle with oil and top with minced garlic. Sprinkle with topping of choice. Place baking sheet one rack down from top rack and broil for 2–4 minutes, until cheese melts and bread is crispy.

Note: Watch closely—it can go from delicious to burnt in the space of a minute.

Mozzarella Topping
1   cup shredded part-skim mozzarella cheese

¼   cup grated Parmesan cheese

1   teaspoon Italian seasoning

¼   teaspoon paprika

Sun-dried Tomato Topping
1   cup shredded part-skim mozzarella cheese

¼   cup grated Parmesan cheese

¼   cup sun-dried tomatoes (in oil), drained and chopped

After removing from oven, garnish with:

2   tablespoons chopped fresh basil

Kalamata and Feta Topping
4   oz. feta cheese, crumbled

16–20 kalamata olives, pitted and halved

1   teaspoon dried oregano

Makes 8 crostini

Phyllo Triangles—Three Ways

When working with phyllo dough, it's important to keep the sheets you are not working with at the moment covered with damp paper towels so the dough does not dry out. Working with phyllo dough is like working a production line. It requires that all other ingredients are prepared before you remove the first sheet of dough from its package. Phyllo triangles can be made ahead and then frozen (uncovered on a baking sheet for 1 hour) and placed in a freezer-safe bag. Bake as directed without thawing.

        Filling of choice from below

12   sheets frozen phyllo dough, thawed according to package directions

⅓   cup butter/canola oil blend, melted

◉ Heat oven to 375°F. Combine ingredients for filling of choice and set aside.

◉ Coat a baking sheet with vegetable spray and set aside. Remove one sheet of phyllo dough to a work surface and brush lightly with melted butter. Place a second sheet of phyllo dough on top and again brush lightly with melted butter. Cut the sheets (lengthwise) into 4 strips. Place one rounded teaspoonful of desired filling at one end of each strip. Fold one corner of the strip over filling diagonally to form a triangle. Continue folding in this diagonal pattern to the end of the strip.

◉ Repeat with remaining strips and place on prepared baking sheet. Repeat with remaining phyllo and filling. Brush tops of triangles lightly with melted butter. Bake for 12–15, minutes until golden brown.

Sausage and Cheddar Filling
½   pound Breakfast Sausage (pg. 117), cooked and drained
½   cup shredded 2% sharp Cheddar cheese (or full-fat for lower lactose)
¼   cup diced onion (about ½ small onion)

Spinach and Feta Filling
1   10-oz. package frozen chopped spinach, thawed and squeezed dry
8   oz. feta cheese, crumbled
1   teaspoon minced garlic (about 2 medium cloves)

Spinach and Sun-dried Tomato Filling
1   10-oz. package frozen chopped spinach, thawed and squeezed dry
½   cup sun-dried tomatoes (in oil or reconstituted in water), drained and chopped
½   cup grated Parmesan cheese
½   teaspoon dried basil

Makes 24 appetizers

Organic Foods

Organic foods are becoming increasingly popular among those concerned about pesticide use on fruits and vegetables, antibiotics and hormones in meat and the environment in general. Consider these points to decide if organic foods are for you:

- Organic foods are grown without pesticides or other chemicals. Natural weed and insect controls are used.

- Organic foods are grown using environmentally friendly methods such as crop rotation and natural fertilizers (manure and composting).

- Organic farming is not a new idea—it is a very old one.

- Organic farming is labor-intensive, and crop yields are lower than commercial farming. This accounts for the higher price and limited selection at the grocery store. Local farmer's markets can be an ideal spot to find organic foods.

- Organic foods have a shorter shelf life and can contain harmful bacteria and other organisms.

- Organic foods may be less attractive and blemished.

- Organic meat is free of antibiotics and hormones. It is also difficult to find and costly.

- The nutritional value of fruits and vegetables is practically the same whether grown organically or not.

- To determine if produce is organic or not, look at the PLU (Price Look Up) number on the label. If it has 4 digits (2345), it is not organic. If it has a 9 in front (92345), it is organic. If it has an 8 in front (82345), it has been genetically altered.

- For more information, visit the Environmental Working Group at www.foodnews.org.

Spicy Beef and Bean Chili

Traditional garnishes of shredded sharp Cheddar and sour cream compliment the spiciness of this dish. If you prefer a milder chili, you can reduce the quantity of the optional ingredients or eliminate them completely. Saltine crackers or crusty bread are a must!

1½	lbs. lean hamburger
1	cup diced onion (about 1 medium onion)
1	cup diced green bell pepper (about 1 medium pepper)
¼	cup sliced pickled jalapeño peppers (optional)
1	14½-oz. can diced tomatoes
1	8-oz. can tomato sauce
1	15-oz. can red kidney or Great Northern beans, rinsed and drained
2	teaspoons chili powder
½	teaspoon cumin
¼	teaspoon coriander
¼	teaspoon crushed red pepper (optional)
¼	teaspoon salt
2–3	dashes hot sauce (optional)
	Shredded Cheddar cheese (optional)
	Lite sour cream or plain yogurt (optional)

◉ In a Dutch oven, cook hamburger, onion, bell pepper, and jalapeños over medium-high heat until hamburger is browned and vegetables are tender, about 10 minutes. Add tomatoes, tomato sauce, beans, chili powder, cumin, coriander, red pepper, salt, and hot sauce and stir thoroughly. Bring to a boil, reduce heat, and simmer 20 minutes.

◉ Garnish with shredded Cheddar cheese and lite sour cream or plain yogurt, if desired.

Makes 6–8 servings

Chicken Chili

2	tablespoons olive oil
1	cup diced onion (about 1 medium onion)
1	cup diced green or red bell pepper (about 1 medium pepper)
¼	cup sliced pickled jalapeño peppers (optional)
2	14½-oz. cans diced tomatoes
2	15-oz. cans kidney, pinto, or black beans (or any combination), rinsed and drained
1	teaspoon chicken base* dissolved in 1 cup of water or 1 cup chicken broth
2½–3	cups roughly chopped, cooked chicken
1½	teaspoons chili powder
½	teaspoon cumin
½	teaspoon coriander
¼	teaspoon salt
¼	teaspoon poultry seasoning
⅛	teaspoon cayenne (optional)
⅛	teaspoon black pepper
	Lite sour cream or plain yogurt (optional)

◉ Heat olive oil over medium-high heat in a Dutch oven. Sauté onion and bell pepper about 5 minutes, until onion is translucent. Add remaining ingredients except sour cream and stir thoroughly. Bring to a boil, reduce heat, and simmer 20 minutes.

◉ Garnish with a dollop of lite sour cream or plain yogurt, if desired.

*Chicken base can be found in the canned soup section of your grocery store, usually stocked near broths and bouillon. Bases give an incredible depth of flavor to dishes and are also available in vegetable, beef, and ham varieties. My favorite brand is Better Than Bouillon because it has few additives or preservatives and no MSG (monosodium glutamate).

Makes 6–8 servings

Venison Chili

2	tablespoons olive oil
1	pound venison loin or stew meat, trimmed and cut into 1½-inch cubes
1	cup diced onion (about 1 medium onion)
1	14½-oz. can beef broth
1	4-oz. can diced green chili peppers
2	tablespoons sliced pickled jalapeño peppers (optional)
1	14½-oz. can diced tomatoes
1	8-oz. can tomato sauce
1	15-oz. can Great Northern beans, rinsed and drained
2	teaspoons chili powder
½	teaspoon cumin
¼	teaspoon coriander
¼	teaspoon salt
	Lite sour cream or plain yogurt (optional)

- Heat oil over medium-high heat in a Dutch oven. Add venison and onion and cook about 5–7 minutes, until meat is brown and onion is translucent.

- Add broth and bring to a boil. Reduce heat, cover, and simmer 1 hour to 1 hour and 15 minutes, until venison is fork-tender.

- Add remaining ingredients except sour cream and stir thoroughly. Bring back to a boil, reduce heat, and simmer 20 minutes.

- Garnish with a dollop of lite sour cream or plain yogurt, if desired.

Makes 6 servings

Creamed Corn Chowder

4	slices center-cut bacon
$\frac{1}{2}$	cup diced onion (about 1 small onion)
1	cup diced celery (about 2 ribs)
1	cup diced carrots (about 2 medium carrots)
2	cups peeled and diced all-purpose or Yukon Gold potatoes (about 2 medium)
1	14$\frac{1}{2}$-oz. can chicken broth
2	14$\frac{1}{2}$-oz. cans creamed corn
$\frac{1}{2}$	teaspoon salt
$\frac{1}{4}$	teaspoon black pepper
$\frac{1}{4}$	teaspoon dried thyme
$\frac{3}{4}$	cup fat-free half and half or chicken broth (optional)*

• Cook bacon in a Dutch oven over medium heat until crisp. Remove bacon and drain on paper towels. Add onion and celery to bacon drippings and cook about 5–7 minutes, until onion is translucent. Add carrots, potatoes, and broth and bring to a boil. Cover and cook about 10 minutes, until vegetables are tender.

• Add corn and seasonings and heat through. At this point the chowder will be very thick. (*If you like a thinner chowder, add either fat-free half and half or chicken broth and simmer for 2 minutes.) Crumble bacon and add back to chowder.

Variations
Chicken Corn Chowder: Add 2 cups roughly chopped cooked chicken with the corn.
Baby Clam Corn Chowder: Add 2 10-oz. cans whole baby clams and substitute crushed red pepper for the thyme.

Makes 6–8 servings

Minestrone

1	tablespoon olive oil
2	cups diced onion (about 1 large onion)
1	cup diced celery (about 2 ribs)
1	cup diced carrots (about 2 medium carrots)
1	small zucchini, ends trimmed, cut lengthwise, and sliced (about 1 cup)
1	teaspoon minced garlic (about 2 cloves)
2	14½-oz. cans beef broth
1	14½-oz. can diced tomatoes
1	teaspoon Italian seasoning
½	teaspoon salt
¼	teaspoon black pepper
1	15-oz. can Great Northern beans, rinsed and drained
1	15-oz. can garbanzo beans, rinsed and drained
1	cup uncooked elbow macaroni
2	cups fresh baby spinach
	Grated Parmesan cheese (optional)

◉ Heat oil in a Dutch oven over medium heat. Add onion, celery, and carrots and cook about 5–7 minutes, until onion is translucent. Add zucchini and cook another 3 minutes. Add garlic and cook 1 minute more.

◉ Add broth, tomatoes, Italian seasoning, salt, and pepper and bring to a boil. Reduce heat, cover, and simmer about 20 minutes.

◉ Add Great Northern beans, garbanzo beans, and macaroni and bring back to a boil. Reduce heat, cover, and simmer about 10–15 minutes, until macaroni is tender. Add spinach and heat through just enough to wilt the spinach.

◉ Ladle into bowls and garnish with grated Parmesan cheese, if desired.

Makes 6–8 servings

Great Northern Bean Soup

1	tablespoon olive oil
1	cup diced onion (about 1 medium onion)
1	cup diced celery (about 2 ribs)
1	cup sliced carrots (about 2 medium carrots)
2	14½-oz. cans chicken broth
3	15-oz. cans Great Northern beans, rinsed and drained
1	10-oz. can chicken breast meat (optional)
2	bay leaves
1	teaspoon Liquid Smoke*
½	teaspoon salt
½	teaspoon dried thyme
¼	teaspoon black pepper

◉ Heat oil in a Dutch oven over medium heat. Add onion, celery, and carrots and cook about 7 minutes, until onion is translucent.

◉ Add remaining ingredients and stir thoroughly. Bring to a boil, reduce heat, cover, and simmer 25–30 minutes, stirring occasionally. Discard bay leaves before serving.

Note: Liquid Smoke adds a woodsy smoke flavor and aroma to foods and contains no additives or preservatives. It can usually be found in the herb and spice section or the condiment section of your grocery store.

Makes 6–8 servings

Earthy Black Bean Soup

2	slices center-cut bacon
2	teaspoons olive oil
1	cup diced onion (about 1 medium onion)
½	cup diced celery (about 1 rib)
2	14½-oz. cans chicken broth
2	15-oz. cans black beans, rinsed and drained
1	10-oz. can chicken breast, drained (optional)
2	bay leaves
½	teaspoon salt
½	teaspoon cumin
½	teaspoon coriander
¼	teaspoon black pepper
¼	teaspoon paprika
	Lite sour cream or plain yogurt (optional)

◉ Cook bacon in a Dutch oven over medium heat until crisp. Remove bacon and drain on paper towels.

◉ Add olive oil, onion, and celery to bacon drippings and cook 5–7 minutes, until onion is translucent.

◉ Add broth, beans, chicken, bay leaves, salt, cumin, coriander, black pepper, and paprika; stir well and bring to a boil. Reduce heat, cover, and simmer 25–30 minutes, stirring occasionally. Discard bay leaves before serving.

◉ Ladle into individual serving bowls and garnish with a dollop of sour cream or plain yogurt and top with crumbled bacon.

Makes 6 servings

Smoky Split Pea Soup

1	pound dried split peas, rinsed and picked over
2	14½-oz. cans chicken broth
4	cups water
1	cup diced onions (about 1 medium onion)
1	cup sliced celery (about 2 ribs)
1½	cups sliced carrots (about 3 medium carrots)
2	bay leaves
1	teaspoon Liquid Smoke*
¾	teaspoon salt
¼	teaspoon black pepper
¼	teaspoon dried thyme

- Combine split peas, broth, and water in a Dutch oven and bring to a boil. Reduce heat, cover, and simmer 1 hour, stirring occasionally.

- Add remaining ingredients and return to a boil. Reduce heat, cover, and simmer 30–40 minutes, stirring occasionally, until vegetables are tender. Discard bay leaves before serving.

If you are not familiar with Liquid Smoke, please see description under Great Northern Bean Soup (pg. 42)

Makes 6 servings

French Onion Soup

1	tablespoon butter/canola oil blend
4	cups thinly sliced onions (about 4 medium onions)
2	14½-oz. cans beef broth
2	teaspoons Worcestershire sauce
¼	teaspoon black pepper
4	slices French or rustic bread
4	slices Swiss or aged Provolone cheese (about 4 ounces)
4	teaspoons grated Parmesan cheese

◉ Melt butter in a Dutch oven over medium heat. Add onions and cook about 10 minutes. Reduce heat to low and cook, stirring occasionally, for another 30 minutes, until the onions are very golden.

◉ Add broth, Worcestershire sauce, and pepper and bring to a boil. Reduce heat and simmer 20 minutes.

◉ Preheat broiler. Arrange bread slices on foil-covered baking sheet. Top each bread slice with 1 slice of cheese and 1 teaspoon Parmesan cheese. Broil for about 2 minutes, until cheese has melted and is golden.

◉ Ladle soup into 4 individual bowls and top each with 1 slice of the toasty cheese bread.

Makes 4 servings

Vegetable Beef Soup

1   tablespoon canola oil

1–1¼ pounds boneless beef chuck or round roast, trimmed and cut
        into 1-inch cubes

2   cups diced onion (about 1 large onion)

2   14½-oz. cans beef broth

2   bay leaves

1   teaspoon Worcestershire sauce

1   teaspoon salt

1   teaspoon herbes de Provence

½   teaspoon black pepper

2   cups sliced carrots (about 4 medium carrots)

1½   cups sliced celery (about 3 ribs)

1   14½-oz. can diced tomatoes

◉ Heat oil in a Dutch oven over medium-high heat. Add beef and cook 5–7 minutes, until browned. Add onion and cook about 5 minutes, until onion is translucent. Add broth, bay leaves, Worcestershire sauce, salt, herbes de Provence, and black pepper and bring to a boil. Reduce heat, cover and simmer, stirring occasionally, 1 hour to 1 hour and 15 minutes, until beef is tender.

◉ Add carrots, celery, and tomatoes and bring to a boil. Reduce heat, cover, and simmer, stirring occasionally, about 30 minutes, until vegetables are tender. Remove bay leaves before serving.

Variation
Vegetable Beef and Barley Soup: Add ½ cup uncooked barley along with the diced tomatoes.

Makes 6–8 servings

Elegant Crab Soup

This recipe is not low lactose—you might consider taking a lactase tablet before consuming.

4	teaspoons butter/canola oil blend
½	cup minced onion (about 1 small onion)
½	cup diced celery (about 1 rib)
½	cup grated carrot (about 1 medium carrot)
1	tablespoon all-purpose flour
1	14½-oz. can chicken broth
2	cups fat-free half and half
½	cup 2% milk
1	bay leaf
2	teaspoons Old Bay seasoning
½	teaspoon salt
¼	teaspoon cayenne pepper (optional)
¼	cup sherry
1	pound lump crabmeat, picked over

◉ Melt butter in a Dutch oven over medium heat. Add onion, celery, and carrot and cook, stirring occasionally, about 7–8 minutes, until vegetables are tender.

◉ Sprinkle with flour and stir well to combine. Whisk in broth until smooth. Add half and half and milk and bring to a simmer. Add bay leaf, Old Bay seasoning, salt, and cayenne pepper, if desired. Simmer about 15–20 minutes, stirring occasionally, until thickened.

◉ Add sherry and crabmeat and simmer another 5 minutes, stirring occasionally. Discard bay leaf before serving.

Makes 6 servings

Chicken Vegetable Soup

Chicken soup is the ultimate comfort food. It is easy to digest and warms the heart as well as the soul by restoring nutrients to the body. This soup is just as delicious when made using a leftover roasted chicken (maybe even better!). Simply reduce initial simmering time to 30 minutes instead of 1 hour.

1	2½- to 3-pound whole chicken, cut up
3	bay leaves
1	teaspoon poultry seasoning
1	teaspoon Italian seasoning
1	teaspoon chicken base (optional)*
2	cups diced onion (about 1 large onion)
1½	cups sliced celery (about 3 ribs, with leaves if possible)
2½	cups sliced carrots (about 5 medium carrots)
3	cups peeled and diced all-purpose or Yukon Gold potatoes (about 3 large)
½	teaspoon salt
¼	teaspoon black pepper

◉ Place chicken pieces in a Dutch oven and add enough water to cover. Add bay leaves, poultry seasoning, and Italian seasoning and bring to a boil. Reduce heat (do not cover) and simmer for 1 hour.

◉ Remove chicken from broth and set aside to cool. Skim fat from broth. Add chicken base to broth if desired. Add onion, celery, carrots, potatoes, salt, and pepper and bring to a boil. Reduce heat (do not cover) and simmer about 25–30 minutes, until vegetables are tender.

◉ When chicken is cool enough to handle, remove skin and bones. Rough chop the chicken meat, add back to soup, and heat through. Discard bay leaves before serving.

* See note about chicken base listed under Chicken Chili (pg. 38).

Variations

Chicken with Rice Soup: Omit potatoes. After adding vegetables to soup, prepare 1 recipe Plain Rice (pg. 184). To serve, spoon ⅓–½ cup rice into soup bowl and ladle 1 cup of soup on top of rice.

Chicken Noodle Soup: Omit potatoes. When vegetables are tender, add 2 cups uncooked fine egg noodles, broken up spaghetti, or other small, shaped pasta. Simmer another 5–10 minutes, until pasta is tender.

Makes 8–10 servings

Poultry Seasoning

2	tablespoons dried sage
1	tablespoon dried thyme
1	teaspoon dried rosemary
1	teaspoon garlic powder
1	teaspoon onion powder
⅛	teaspoon cayenne

◉ Mix ingredients together and store in an airtight container.

Makes about ¼ cup

Creamy Mushroom Soup

2	teaspoons butter/canola oil blend
1	cup diced onion (about 1 medium onion)
1	cup diced celery (about 2 ribs)
1	pound white or cremini mushrooms, stems removed and caps sliced
1	14½-oz. can chicken broth
½	teaspoon salt
¼	teaspoon black pepper
1½	cups fat-free half and half or soy milk
2	tablespoons all-purpose flour

◉ Melt butter in a Dutch oven over medium heat. Add onion and celery and cook about 5–7 minutes, until tender.

◉ Add mushrooms, broth, salt, and pepper and bring to a boil. Reduce heat, cover, and simmer about 10–12 minutes, until mushrooms are tender.

◉ In a lidded jar, shake together the half and half and flour until blended. Whisk half and half and flour mixture into soup in a slow, steady stream. Cook, stirring constantly, about 2–3 minutes, until thick and creamy—do not boil.

Makes 4 servings

Carrot, Potato, and Leek Soup

2	teaspoons butter/canola oil blend
2	leeks (white part only), diced
1	cup diced onion (about 1 medium onion)
2	14½-oz. cans chicken broth
3	cups thinly sliced carrots (about 6 medium)
3	cups peeled and diced all-purpose potatoes (about 3 large)
1	bay leaf
½	teaspoon salt
½	teaspoon dried thyme
¼	teaspoon black pepper
1	cup frozen peas (optional)

◉ Melt butter in a Dutch oven over medium heat. Add leeks and onion and cook about 5–7 minutes, until tender.

◉ Add broth, carrots, potatoes, bay leaf, salt, thyme, and pepper and bring to a boil. Reduce heat, cover, and simmer about 25–30 minutes, until vegetables are tender. Add peas, if desired, and cook another 5 minutes. Remove bay leaf before serving.

Makes 4–6 servings

Skimming Fat from Broth

There are several methods to skim the fat from broth.

◉ Lay paper towels gently on top of broth and remove carefully—repeat several times.

◉ Place an ice cube in dampened cheesecloth and run it along the top of broth. The fat will congeal on contact with the ice.

◉ Use a large metal spoon and gently skim fat that rises to top.

◉ Use a meat baster (bulb baster) to suck up the fat.

◉ Use a fat-separating pitcher that is specially designed to allow you to pour off the broth while the fat stays in the pitcher.

◉ Use an oil mop (fat mop/grease mop). These are made of plastic that sops up the fat but not the broth.

◉ Cool broth and refrigerate for 6–8 hours. Spoon off solidified fat.

Simple Salad 101

6   cups varietal lettuce, washed and torn into bite-sized pieces

Choose one or any combination:

      Baby greens, radicchio, red or green leaf, Bibb, romaine, iceberg, Boston, spinach

¼   cup cider vinegar

1   tablespoon sugar

◉ Place prepared lettuce in a large bowl. Drizzle with vinegar, sprinkle with sugar, and toss to coat. Serve immediately.

Makes 4 servings

Simple Salad 102

Before varietal lettuce was widely available and salads prepared with them were in vogue, the iceberg wedge was very popular.

1   large head of iceberg lettuce

◉ Core, remove outer leaves, and rinse the head of lettuce in cold water. Chill 1–2 hours to crisp.

◉ Cut into 6 wedges and drizzle each wedge with 2 tablespoons of your favorite salad dressing. Thousand Island (pg. 69), Buttermilk Herb (pg. 66), and Green Goddess (pg. 68) are all good choices, as are vinaigrettes (pg. 70).

Makes 6 servings

Greek Salad

Feta cheese is very strong in flavor, and a little goes a long way. Even if you are lactose intolerant, you may be able to tolerate the small amount of feta in this recipe. If you prefer, you can substitute cubed sharp Cheddar or grated Parmesan cheese.

½	large head iceberg lettuce, cored, outer leaves removed, and rinsed
½	head romaine lettuce, ribs removed and rinsed
1	small red onion, sliced thin
1	small cucumber, peeled and sliced
12	kalamata olives, pitted and halved
2	ounces crumbled feta cheese
¼	cup Greek Vinaigrette (pg. 70)
1	Roma tomato, seeded and cut into quarters

◉ Tear iceberg and romaine lettuce into bite-sized pieces and place in large bowl. Add onion, cucumber, olives, and feta cheese. Drizzle with vinaigrette and toss to coat.

◉ Divide among 4 salad plates and garnish with tomato wedge. Serve immediately.

Makes 4 servings

Traditional Caesar Salad

1   head romaine lettuce, ribs removed, rinsed, and torn into bite-sized pieces

1½   tablespoons fresh lemon juice (about ½ of a fresh lemon)

¼   teaspoon salt

3   anchovy fillets or 1 teaspoon anchovy paste

1½   teaspoons minced garlic (about 3 medium cloves)

2   teaspoons Dijon mustard or 1 teaspoon dry mustard

1   egg yolk*

¼   cup olive oil

¼   cup grated Parmesan cheese

2   cups Seasoned Croutons (pg. 57)

◉ Prepare romaine and place in a large bowl. Drizzle with lemon juice and toss lightly.

◉ In a small bowl combine salt, anchovy fillets or paste, and minced garlic and mash together with fork. Stir in mustard and mix well. Stir in egg yolk* and mix well. Whisk in olive oil in a slow steady stream until fully incorporated.

◉ Drizzle romaine with dressing. Sprinkle with Parmesan cheese and toss well. Top with croutons and serve immediately.

If you are concerned about using raw egg yolk, substitute 1 hard-boiled egg yolk, mashed.

Makes 4 servings

Caesar on the Lam

1	1-lb. bag prewashed and torn romaine lettuce
¼	cup Marie's Caesar dressing*
¼	cup grated Parmesan cheese
2	cups packaged croutons

◉ Place romaine, Caesar dressing, and Parmesan cheese in large bowl and toss well to coat. Top with croutons and serve immediately.

* *Marie's brand salad dressings are very flavorful, contain no preservatives, and are available in the refrigerated salad dressing section of your local grocery store.*

Makes 4 servings

Seasoned Croutons

1	tablespoon butter/canola oil blend
1	baguette or rustic bread, cut into 1½- to 2-inch cubes (about 4–5 cups)
2	tablespoons olive oil
1	teaspoon Italian seasoning
½	teaspoon garlic powder
¼	teaspoon onion powder
¼	teaspoon salt
⅛	teaspoon black pepper

◉ Preheat oven to 375°F. Coat a baking sheet with vegetable spray.

◉ Melt the butter in a skillet over medium heat. Add bread cubes and drizzle with olive oil. Sprinkle with seasonings and toss well to coat. Spread seasoned bread cubes in a single layer on prepared baking sheet.

◉ Bake 10 minutes, stir croutons, and bake another 5–10 minutes, until golden and crispy. Cool to room temperature. Croutons will last about 1 week in an airtight container.

Makes about 4 cups

Cucumber Salad

4 cups peeled, seeded, and thinly sliced cucumbers (about 4 medium cucumbers)

1 cup thinly sliced Vidalia or red onion

½ cup cider vinegar

2 tablespoons sugar

½ teaspoon salt

½ teaspoon black pepper

◉ Combine all ingredients in a medium bowl and toss well to coat. Cover and chill at least 2 hours or overnight.

Variations
Balsamic Cucumber Salad: Substitute balsamic vinegar for the cider vinegar.
Roma and Cucumber Salad: Add 2–3 sliced Roma tomatoes.
Cucumber Salad with Dill: Add 1 tablespoon chopped fresh dill.

Makes 6 servings

Summer Fruit Salad with Lime Dressing

3–4   tablespoons fresh lime juice (about 2 medium limes)

2   tablespoons sugar

½   seedless watermelon, cut into bite-sized pieces

1   medium cantaloupe, cut into bite-sized pieces

2   large peaches, pitted, peeled, and sliced

1   cup seedless red or white grapes, halved

1   pint strawberries, stems removed and halved

1   pint blueberries

½   pint raspberries

Fresh mint (optional)

◉ Stir together lime juice and sugar and set aside. Combine all the fruits in a large bowl. Drizzle with lime dressing and toss gently. Cover and chill 1–2 hours before serving. Garnish with fresh mint, if desired.

Makes 12–14 cups

Three-Bean Salad

Fresh green beans give this traditional salad a brightness both in color and in flavor that just can't be matched by canned beans. If they are not in season, you can substitute frozen green beans cooked according to package directions.

1	pound fresh green beans, ends trimmed
1	15-oz. can black beans, rinsed and drained
1	15-oz. can pinto beans, rinsed and drained
½	cup thinly sliced onion (about 1 small onion)
¼	cup Basic Vinaigrette (pg. 70)

◉ Place green beans in a Dutch oven with 2 inches of water. Cover, bring to a boil, and cook about 10–12 minutes, until tender. Remove green beans to a bowl of ice water to stop the cooking process. Drain green beans and place in bowl.

◉ Add remaining ingredients and toss to coat. Cover and chill 2 hours before serving.

Makes 6–8 servings

Sun-Dried Tomato and Mozzarella Salad

My apologies to those who are lactose intolerant. There simply is no substitution for the fresh mozzarella in this recipe.

4	cups salad greens, torn into bite-sized pieces
¼	cup thinly sliced red onion (about ½ small onion)
8–10	sun-dried tomato halves (not packed in oil), reconstituted, drained, and sliced
6	ounces fresh mozzarella, cubed
2	tablespoons olive oil
2	tablespoons red wine vinegar
¼	cup fresh basil, torn
1	teaspoon Italian seasoning
½	teaspoon salt
¼	teaspoon black pepper

◉ Place prepared greens and onion in a large bowl. In a medium bowl combine remaining ingredients and toss well to coat; add to salad greens and toss well. Serve immediately.

Makes 4 servings

Deluxe Pasta Salad

8   ounces bowtie or shell pasta, cooked to package directions

¼   cup diced red onion (about ½ small onion)

½   cup diced celery (about 1 rib)

1   small zucchini, cut in half lengthwise and sliced

1   7-oz. jar roasted red pepper, drained and chopped

8–10 sun-dried tomatoes (not packed in oil), reconstituted, drained, and sliced

8–10 kalamata olives, pitted and halved

⅓   cup Basic Vinaigrette (pg. 70)

◉ Prepare pasta and drain. Combine all ingredients in a large bowl and toss to coat evenly. Cover and chill at least 2 hours before serving.

Makes 6–8 servings

Best Potato Salad Ever

Yes, I said it: This is the best potato salad ever! It is the perfect side dish for sandwiches, hamburgers and back yard barbeques. It is also one of those dishes that is even better the second day (if it lasts that long). This recipe can be easily doubled if feeding a larger group. Please note that it is important to allow potatoes to cool properly so they will retain their shape when cubed.

2	pounds all-purpose potatoes (about 6 medium potatoes)
¼	teaspoon salt
3	hard-boiled eggs, coarsely chopped
½	cup diced onion (about 1 small onion)
1	cup diced celery (about 2 ribs)
½	cup Miracle Whip
1	teaspoon prepared mustard
½	teaspoon salt
¼	teaspoon black pepper
¼	teaspoon paprika

◎ Wash potatoes, cut in half, and place in a medium saucepan. Cover potatoes with water and add ¼ teaspoon salt. Bring to a boil and cook until fork-tender, about 25 minutes. Drain and cool to room temperature.

◎ When potatoes have cooled, peel and cube them and place in a large bowl. Add eggs, onion, celery, Miracle Whip, mustard, ½ teaspoon salt, and pepper and toss gently to coat. Transfer to a clean serving bowl if desired and sprinkle with paprika. Cover and chill at least 2 hours before serving.

Variations
Best Red Potato Salad Ever: Substitute red potatoes for the all-purpose but do not peel them. Add 1 tablespoon prepared horseradish.

Makes 6 servings

Seafood Pasta Salad

This is an adaptation of a recipe given to me by Danny O'Rourk who, along with his wife Cindy, owned the Sunset Caye Yacht Club in Folly Beach, South Carolina. I had the pleasure of working at the restaurant for more than five years. When in season, the shrimp and crabs came straight off the boat the same day they were caught. This was amazing to me, a Yankee from northern New York State! The staff and the regulars at "The Marina" became a second family to me, and I cherish the memories made there.

1	pound shell pasta, cooked to package directions
2	tablespoons butter/canola oil blend
8	ounces fresh large shrimp, peeled, deveined, and tails removed
8	ounces fresh sea scallops
8	ounces lump crabmeat, picked over
1½	cups diced celery (about 3 ribs)
6	green onions, sliced thin
½	cup diced green bell pepper (about ½ medium pepper)
½	cup diced red bell pepper (about ½ medium pepper)
1	cup Miracle Whip
2	teaspoons Old Bay seasoning
1	teaspoon Italian seasoning
½	teaspoon garlic powder
½	teaspoon salt
½	teaspoon black pepper

◉ Prepare pasta and drain. Melt butter in skillet over medium heat. Add shrimp, scallops, and crab and sauté until shrimp turn pink and scallops are opaque, about 3–5 minutes.

◉ Remove from skillet to a platter to cool. Combine pasta, seafood, and remaining ingredients in a large bowl and toss gently to coat. Cover and chill at least 2 hours or overnight.

Makes 8–10 servings

Tossed Salad Combos

Here are a few ideas to give an ordinary tossed salad fresh appeal.

Baby spinach
Sliced peaches
Sliced green onions
Blue Cheese Dressing (pg. 66)

Baby spinach
Sliced cremini mushrooms
Sliced red onion
Balsamic Vinaigrette (pg. 70)

Baby spinach
Chopped, cooked chicken breast meat
Raspberries
Sliced sweet onion
Raspberry Vinaigrette (pg. 70)

Baby spinach
Sliced red onion
Fresh or frozen blueberries
Crumbled feta cheese
Balsamic Vinaigrette (pg. 70)

Romaine
Boston lettuce
Sliced red onion
Chopped hard-boiled egg
Russian Dressing (pg. 69)

Green leaf lettuce
Iceberg lettuce
Sliced black olives
Crumbled feta cheese
Creamy Cucumber Dressing (pg. 68)

Mixed salad greens
Sliced sweet onion
Sliced deli turkey
Shredded sharp Cheddar cheese
1000 Island Dressing (pg. 69)
Top with croutons

Mixed salad greens
Sliced Roma tomatoes
Frozen peas, thawed
Sliced white mushrooms
Basic Vinaigrette (pg. 70)
Top with crumbled bacon

Bibb lettuce
Iceberg lettuce
Sliced Roma tomatoes
Buttermilk Herb Dressing (pg. 66)
Top with crumbled bacon and croutons

Mixed salad greens
Sliced deli turkey ham
Sliced Swiss cheese
Honey-Dijon Dressing (pg. 67)
Top with croutons

Boston lettuce
Red leaf lettuce
Peeled and sliced cucumbers
Alfalfa sprouts
Green Goddess Dressing (pg. 68)

Buttermilk Herb Dressing

¾ cup buttermilk*

½ cup Miracle Whip

¼ cup reduced-fat sour cream or plain yogurt

1 teaspoon dried parsley

1 teaspoon Italian seasoning

¾ teaspoon onion powder

¾ teaspoon garlic powder

¼ teaspoon salt

¼ teaspoon black pepper

Whisk all ingredients together in a bowl. Cover and chill.

Tip: If you don't have buttermilk on hand, place 1 tablespoon white vinegar or lemon juice in a measuring cup and add enough milk to equal 1 cup. Allow to stand 5 minutes.

Variation
Blue Cheese Dressing: Omit onion and garlic powders and add 4 ounces crumbled blue cheese.

Makes about 1½ cups

Honey-Dijon Dressing

¾   cup reduced-fat sour cream or plain yogurt

¼   cup Dijon mustard

¼   cup honey

1   tablespoon cider vinegar

Whisk all ingredients together in a bowl. Cover and chill.

Variation
Maple-Dijon Dressing: Substitute pure maple syrup for the honey.

Makes about 1 ¼ cups

Green Goddess Dressing

½	cup loosely packed fresh flat-leaf parsley
½	cup Miracle Whip
¼	cup reduced-fat sour cream or plain yogurt
1	tablespoon red wine vinegar
1	tablespoon fresh lemon juice (about ½ small lemon)
1	teaspoon anchovy paste
¼	teaspoon black pepper
⅛	teaspoon dried tarragon

◉ Combine all ingredients in a food processor or blender and process until smooth. Cover and chill.

Makes about 1¼ cups

Creamy Cucumber Dressing

¾–1	cup peeled, seeded, and finely diced cucumber (about 1 medium cucumber)
⅓	cup Miracle Whip
⅓	cup reduced-fat sour cream or plain yogurt
2	tablespoons fresh chives, snipped
¼	teaspoon salt

◉ Whisk all ingredients together in a bowl. Cover and chill.

Makes about 1½ cups

Russian Dressing

¾   cup Miracle Whip

¼   cup ketchup

¼   cup dill pickle relish

1   teaspoon fresh lemon juice

¼   teaspoon onion powder

¼   teaspoon salt

⅛   teaspoon black pepper

◉ Whisk all ingredients together in a bowl. Cover and chill.

Makes about 1¼ cups

1000 Island Dressing

This dressing became famous after George Boldt, owner/manager of the Waldorf-Astoria Hotel, ordered that it be put on the hotel menu. He was given the recipe while constructing Boldt Castle, a gift to his wife, on Heart Island in the 1000 Islands region of northern New York. This is the area where I was raised, and, in fact, I worked at a resort with a grand view of the castle for several years.

¾   cup Miracle Whip

¼   cup ketchup

¼   cup sweet pickle relish

1   hard-boiled egg, diced

◉ Whisk all ingredients together in a bowl. Cover and chill.

Makes about 1¼ cups

Basic Vinaigrette

⅔   cup olive oil

⅓   cup red wine vinegar

1   tablespoon Italian seasoning

1   teaspoon sugar

½   teaspoon salt

¼   teaspoon black pepper

◉ Combine all ingredients in a lidded jar and shake well. Use immediately or store covered in the refrigerator. Allow to stand at room temperature for 30 minutes after refrigeration, and shake well before serving.

Variations
Balsamic Vinaigrette: Omit sugar and substitute balsamic vinegar for the red wine vinegar.
French Vinaigrette: Substitute herbes de Provence for the Italian seasoning and add ½ teaspoon dry mustard.
Greek Vinaigrette: Substitute dried oregano for the Italian seasoning.
Raspberry Vinaigrette: Omit sugar, substitute balsamic vinegar for the red wine vinegar, and add 3 tablespoons raspberry all-fruit jam.
Signature Vinaigrette: Experiment with flavored oils, cider, or white vinegar, and various dried herbs to create your own signature vinaigrette.

Makes about 1 cup

Deli-Style Tuna Salad

2   6-oz. cans albacore tuna (packed in water), drained*

½   cup finely diced celery (about 1 rib)

¼   cup finely diced onion (about ½ small onion)

2   teaspoons sweet pickle relish (optional)

¼   cup Miracle Whip

◉ Combine all ingredients in a bowl and mix well. Use to make sandwiches or serve with crackers. Best when chilled for at least 1 hour.

If you are concerned about mercury levels in albacore tuna because of pregnancy or if serving to children, substitute chunk light tuna.

Makes about 2 cups

Classic Tuna Melt

1   teaspoon butter/canola blend

2   slices Italian or rustic bread

1   ounce sliced sharp Cheddar or Swiss cheese

½   cup Deli-Style Tuna Salad (pg. 71)

◉ Heat skillet over medium heat. Spread butter on one side of each slice of bread. Lay one bread slice, butter side down, in skillet. Place cheese on bread and top with tuna salad. Place second slice of bread on top of tuna, butter side up. Cook about 3 minutes on each side until golden and cheese has melted.

◉ Cut sandwich in half to serve.

Makes 1 sandwich

Chicken Salad

2–2½ cups chopped cooked chicken or 2 10-oz. cans white meat
      chicken, drained

½   cup finely diced celery (about 1 rib)

¼   cup finely diced onion (about ½ small onion)

1   tablespoon sweet pickle relish

⅓   cup Miracle Whip

¼   teaspoon salt

⅛   teaspoon black pepper

◉ Combine all ingredients in a bowl and mix well. Use to make sandwiches or serve atop a bed of lettuce greens and/or with crackers. Best when chilled for at least 1 hour.

Variation
Turkey Salad: Substitute chopped, cooked turkey for the chicken.

Makes about 3 cups

Avocado BLT

4	slices center-cut bacon
2	tablespoons Miracle Whip
4	slices Italian or rustic bread, toasted
4	whole leaves of Bibb lettuce
1	very ripe avocado, pitted
1	Roma tomato, sliced thin

◉ Cook bacon in skillet over medium-high heat until crisp. Drain on paper towels. Spread 1 tablespoon Miracle Whip on 2 slices of toasted bread. Top each with 2 leaves of Bibb lettuce.

◉ Scoop out avocado halves, move to a cutting board, and cut into 4 slices each. Place avocado slices on top of lettuce. Top with bacon, tomato slices, and remaining slices of toasted bread. Cut each sandwich in half to serve.

Makes 2 sandwiches

Sloppy Joes

Serve these sandwiches with a fresh green salad or a side of potato salad. Don't forget plenty of napkins!

1	pound lean hamburger
1	cup diced onion (about 1 medium onion)
½	cup diced green bell pepper (about ½ medium pepper)
1	8-oz. can tomato sauce
¼	cup ketchup
1	tablespoon Worcestershire sauce
¼	teaspoon garlic powder
⅛	teaspoon onion powder
⅛	teaspoon chili powder
4	toasted sandwich rolls

◉ Cook hamburger, onion, and bell pepper in skillet over medium heat until meat is browned and vegetables are tender, about 7–10 minutes. Add remaining ingredients and bring to a boil.

◉ Reduce heat, cover, and simmer, stirring occasionally, about 15–20 minutes, until thickened. Serve on toasted rolls.

Makes 4 sandwiches

Pulled Pork Sammies

1	2½- to 3-pound boneless pork shoulder roast, trimmed
½	teaspoon salt
¼	teaspoon black pepper
¼	teaspoon onion powder
¼	teaspoon garlic powder
¼	teaspoon poultry seasoning
1	tablespoon canola or olive oil
3	cups water
1	recipe Barbecue Sauce (pg. 190) or 1½ cups bottled barbecue sauce
	Toasted sandwich rolls

◉ Sprinkle roast with salt, pepper, onion powder, garlic powder, and poultry seasoning.

◉ Heat oil in a Dutch oven over medium-high heat. Add roast and brown on all sides. Add water and bring to a boil. Reduce heat, cover, and simmer about 2 hours and 15 minutes to 2 hours and 30 minutes, turning occasionally, until fork-tender.

◉ Remove roast from Dutch oven and allow to cool slightly. Drain any remaining liquid from Dutch oven and use it to prepare barbeque sauce. When pork is cool enough to handle, shred the meat with hands or with a fork. Add to sauce and heat through.

◉ Serve on toasted sandwich rolls.

Makes 8–10 sandwiches

Open-Faced Crab Sammies

Serve a simple green salad with these sandwiches for an elegant lunch.

2   English muffins, split and lightly toasted

1   pound lump crabmeat, picked over

1   cup shredded Swiss cheese (about 4 oz.)

2   tablespoons Miracle Whip

1   tablespoon fresh lemon juice

¼   teaspoon salt

¼   teaspoon Old Bay seasoning

⅛   teaspoon black pepper

1   Roma tomato, ends removed and cut into 4 slices

      Lemon wedges (optional)

◉ Heat oven to broil. Place toasted muffin halves split side up on a baking sheet.

◉ Combine crabmeat, cheese, Miracle Whip, lemon juice, salt, Old Bay seasoning, and pepper in a bowl and mix gently. Top muffin halves with crab mixture. Top each sandwich with a slice of tomato.

◉ Broil 3–4 minutes, until lightly browned. Garnish with lemon wedges, if desired.

Makes 4 sandwiches

Lean Burgers with the Works

Many cooks say the only way to prepare a flavorful burger is to start with 20% fat hamburger. I couldn't disagree more.

1¼	pounds lean hamburger
2	tablespoons Worcestershire sauce, divided
4	slices (about 1 oz. each) sharp Cheddar or Swiss cheese
4	toasted hamburger rolls
8	whole leaves of Bibb lettuce
1	Roma tomato, thinly sliced
¼	cup thinly sliced onion (about ½ small onion)
	Ketchup
	Prepared mustard
	Miracle Whip

◉ Heat skillet over medium-high heat. Gently shape hamburger into 4 equal patties. Place burgers in skillet and drizzle with 1 tablespoon Worcestershire sauce and cook about 4 minutes.

◉ Flip burgers and flatten them with the back side of your spatula. Drizzle with remaining 1 tablespoon Worcestershire sauce and cook another 3–5 minutes, until no longer pink inside. Do not overcook.

◉ Top burgers with cheese slices and allow cheese to melt, about 1–2 minutes.

◉ Serve burgers on toasted rolls and top with lettuce, tomato, onion, and condiments of choice.

Makes 4 sandwiches

Tuna Burgers

2	6-oz. cans albacore tuna* packed in water, drained
½	cup plain bread crumbs
1	egg white
½	cup diced onion (about ½ small)
½	cup diced celery (about 1 rib)
1	teaspoon fresh lemon juice
¼	teaspoon salt
⅛	teaspoon black pepper
1	tablespoon canola oil
4	toasted sandwich rolls
	Tartar Sauce (pg. 189)

◉ In a medium bowl combine tuna, bread crumbs, egg white, onion, celery, lemon juice, salt, and pepper and mix well.

◉ Heat oil in skillet over medium heat. Shape tuna mixture into 4 patties and add to skillet. Cook about 4–5 minutes on each side until golden brown.

◉ Serve on toasted rolls with tartar sauce, if desired.

Variation
Salmon Burgers: Substitute 1 (12 oz.) can pink salmon** or 12 oz. leftover Rosemary and Lemon Salmon (pg. 143) for the tuna.

If concerned about mercury levels in albacore tuna, substitute chunk light tuna.
** *If using canned salmon, increase fresh lemon juice to 2 teaspoons.*

Makes 4 sandwiches

Smoky Black Bean Burgers

1	15-oz. can black beans, rinsed and drained
¼	cup plain bread crumbs
2	tablespoons Miracle Whip
½	teaspoon salt
½	teaspoon chili powder
½	teaspoon cumin
½	teaspoon coriander
1½	tablespoons olive or canola oil
1–2	tablespoons all-purpose flour
4	toasted sandwich rolls
	Fresh Tomato Salsa (pg. 27) or bottled salsa

◉ Mash beans in a medium bowl with potato masher or fork. Add bread crumbs, Miracle Whip, salt, chili powder, cumin, and coriander and mix well. Cover and chill for 30 minutes.

◉ Heat oil in skillet over medium heat. Dust hands with flour and shape bean mixture into 4 patties and place in skillet. Cook patties about 4–5 minutes on each side, until lightly browned. Drain on paper towels.

◉ Serve on toasted rolls with salsa, if desired.

Makes 4 sandwiches

Marinated Portobello Burgers

4	portobello mushrooms, stems removed and caps sliced about ½-inch thick
1	cup Basic Vinaigrette (pg. 70)
1	tablespoon Worcestershire sauce
¼	teaspoon salt
¼	teaspoon black pepper
4	slices aged Provolone cheese (about 1 oz. each)
4	toasted hamburger buns

◉ Place mushroom slices in a ziplock bag. Cover with vinaigrette and Worcestershire sauce. Place in refrigerator and marinate for at least 2 hours.

◉ Heat a skillet over medium heat. Add mushroom slices and discard vinaigrette. Season mushrooms with salt and pepper and cook about 5–7 minutes, until tender.

◉ Top with cheese and allow cheese to melt. Divide among toasted buns to serve.

Makes 4 sandwiches

Hearty Black Bean Burgers with Portobellos and Red Onions

1	15-oz. can black beans, rinsed and drained
¼	cup plain bread crumbs
1	egg
2	tablespoons ketchup
2	tablespoons minced onion
1	teaspoon Worcestershire sauce
½	teaspoon salt
¼	teaspoon black pepper
½	teaspoon garlic powder
3	tablespoons olive or canola oil, divided
1	cup thinly sliced red onion (about 1 medium onion)
2	portobello mushrooms, stems removed and caps sliced about ½-inch thick
1	teaspoon minced garlic (about 2 medium cloves)
1–2	tablespoons all-purpose flour
4	slices sharp Cheddar cheese (about 1-oz. each)
4	toasted hamburger buns
	Ketchup (optional)
	Prepared mustard (optional)

◉ Mash beans in a medium bowl with potato masher or fork. Add bread crumbs, egg, ketchup, minced onion, Worcestershire sauce, salt, pepper, and garlic powder and mix well. Cover and chill.

◉ Heat 1½ tablespoons oil in skillet over medium heat and add red onion and sliced portobellos and sauté about 5–7 minutes, until tender. Add minced garlic and cook 1 minute more. Remove onions and mushrooms from skillet and set aside.

◉ In same skillet, heat remaining 1½ tablespoons oil over medium heat. Dust hands with flour and shape bean mixture into 4 patties and add to skillet. Cook patties about 4–5 minutes on each side until lightly browned.

◉ Top each patty with one-fourth of the mushrooms and onions and then with 1 slice of cheese. Allow cheese to melt.

◉ Serve on toasted buns with ketchup and mustard, if desired.

Makes 4 sandwiches

Italian Sausage Sammies

1	tablespoon olive oil
1	pound Sweet Italian Sausage (pg. 117)
1	cup sliced green or red bell pepper (about 1 medium pepper)
1	cup sliced onion (about 1 medium onion)
4	slices aged Provolone cheese (about 1-oz. each)
4	toasted hoagie rolls
1	cup warmed Marinara Sauce (pg. 163) or bottled sauce
¼	cup grated Parmesan cheese

◉ Heat oil in skillet over medium-high heat. Add sausage, bell pepper, and onion and cook, stirring frequently to break up sausage, about 10–12 minutes, until sausage is browned and vegetables are tender.

◉ Top with cheese and allow cheese to melt. Divide sausage mixture among hoagie rolls. Top each sandwich with ¼ cup marinara sauce and 1 tablespoon Parmesan cheese to serve.

Makes 4 sandwiches

Oatmeal Bread

This bread is slightly sweet and makes excellent sandwiches. If desired, sprinkle top of loaf lightly with oats before baking.

1	package active dry yeast
½	cup warm water (105–115°F)
1	cup scalded 2% milk or soy milk, cooled
¼	cup dark brown sugar
2	tablespoons butter/canola oil blend, softened
1	teaspoon salt
⅛	teaspoon ground nutmeg
1	cup old-fashioned or quick oats
2½	cups unbleached all-purpose flour, plus more for dusting
½	teaspoon olive or canola oil

◉ Dissolve yeast in water and set aside for 5 minutes.

◉ In a large bowl combine scalded milk, brown sugar, butter, salt, and nutmeg and mix well. Add yeast, oats, and 2 cups flour and beat with an electric mixer until smooth. Stir in remaining ½ cup flour.

◉ Turn dough onto floured surface and knead about 7–8 minutes, until smooth and elastic. Place oil in a large clean bowl. Place dough in bowl and turn to coat top. Cover with plastic wrap or clean kitchen towel and let rise until double in bulk, about 1 hour.

◉ Punch down dough and allow to rest 10 minutes.

◉ Coat a loaf pan with vegetable spray. On lightly floured surface, roll dough into a rectangle. Begin at narrow end and roll dough up tightly. Pinch edges to seal. Place seam side down in prepared pan. Cover with plastic wrap or clean kitchen towel and let rise until double in bulk, about 30–40 minutes.

◉ Preheat oven to 400°. Bake for 25–30 minutes, until golden brown and loaf sounds hollow when tapped. Remove immediately from pan and cool on wire rack.

Makes 1 loaf, about 12 servings

No-Knead White Bread

This is about as easy as it gets for preparing white sandwich bread! Not only is it great for sandwiches, it is equally good for making toast and croutons.

½	cup warm water (105–115°F)
1	package active dry yeast
4	teaspoons sugar
½	cup scalded 2% or soy milk, cooled
1½	teaspoons salt
1½	tablespoons butter/canola oil blend
1	large egg
3–3¼	cups unbleached all-purpose flour

◉ Combine water, yeast, and sugar and set aside for 5 minutes until foamy.

◉ In a large bowl combine yeast mixture, scalded milk, salt, butter, egg, and 3 cups of flour and beat with an electric mixer until smooth. Stir in more flour (up to ¼ cup) if necessary to make a stiff (not sticky) dough.

◉ Coat a loaf pan with vegetable spray. On a floured surface, shape dough into loaf and place in prepared pan. Cover with plastic wrap or clean kitchen towel and let rise until double in bulk, about 1 hour.

◉ Preheat oven to 350°F. Bake for 30–35 minutes, until golden and loaf sounds hollow when tapped. Remove from pan immediately and cool on wire rack.

Makes 1 loaf, about 12 servings

English Muffin Bread

This breakfast bread is easy because there's no kneading required. It's delicious when toasted and served with nut butters, spreadable fruit, or honey.

½	cup warm water (105–115°F)
1	package active dry yeast
	Cornmeal for dusting
3¼	cups unbleached all-purpose flour
2	teaspoons sugar
1	teaspoon salt
1	cup scalded 2% milk or soy milk, cooled

◉ Combine water and yeast and set aside for 5 minutes until foamy.

◉ Coat a loaf pan with vegetable spray and sprinkle with cornmeal. In a large bowl combine flour, sugar, and salt.

◉ Add scalded milk and yeast mixture to flour and stir to combine. Place dough in prepared pan and sprinkle with cornmeal. Cover with plastic wrap or clean kitchen towel and let rise until double in bulk, 45 minutes to 1 hour.

◉ Preheat oven to 400°F. Bake about 22–25 minutes, until golden and loaf sounds hollow when tapped. Remove from pan immediately and cool on wire rack.

Makes 1 loaf, about 12 servings

Rosemary Focaccia

Focaccia is a versatile bread. It can be served as an accompaniment with an entrée or salad or used for sandwiches or as a pizza base. With a few simple toppings, it becomes a company-pleasing appetizer.

1	cup warm water (105–115°F)
1	package active dry yeast
1	teaspoon sugar
3½	tablespoons olive oil, divided
1	teaspoon salt
3½	cups unbleached all-purpose flour, plus more for dusting
1½	teaspoons kosher or sea salt
1½	tablespoons chopped fresh rosemary

◉ In a small bowl combine water, yeast, and sugar and set aside for 5 minutes until foamy.

◉ In a large bowl combine 2 tablespoons olive oil, salt, and flour. Stir in yeast mixture until a soft dough forms. Turn dough onto floured surface and knead for about 7–10 minutes—dusting with more flour as needed to keep from sticking—until smooth and elastic.

◉ Place ½ teaspoon olive oil in a large clean bowl. Form dough into a ball, place in oiled bowl, and turn to coat top. Cover with plastic wrap or clean kitchen towel and allow to rise until double in bulk, about 1 hour.

◉ Coat a baking sheet with vegetable spray. Punch down dough and pat into pan. Cover with plastic wrap or clean kitchen towel and let rise until double in bulk, about 30 minutes.

◉ Preheat oven to 425°F. With fingertips, make indentations over surface of dough. Brush or drizzle with remaining 1 tablespoon of olive oil. Sprinkle with salt and rosemary. Bake about 20–25 minutes, until golden.

Variations
Parmesan Focaccia: Omit rosemary. Top with ¼ cup grated Parmesan cheese, 2 medium Roma tomatoes (sliced thin), and 1 teaspoon Italian seasoning.

Roasted Red Pepper Focaccia: Omit rosemary. Top with 1 7-oz. jar roasted red peppers, sliced; ¼ cup sun-dried tomatoes (packed in oil or reconstituted), chopped; and 2 tablespoons sliced fresh basil leaves.

Spinach Focaccia: Omit rosemary. Top with 1 10-oz. package frozen spinach, thawed and squeezed dry; ½ cup thinly sliced red onion, about 1 small onion; and 1 teaspoon garlic powder.

Black Olive Focaccia: Omit rosemary. Top with 18–20 black olives, pitted and halved; 2 ounces crumbled feta cheese; and 1 teaspoon dried oregano.

Pizza Base Focaccia: Omit rosemary. Bake 20 minutes. Top with sauce and favorite pizza toppings. Increase oven temperature to 450°F and bake an additional 12–15 minutes.

Makes 1 flat bread, about 12 servings

Tips on Kneading Bread Dough

- Pulling and pushing bread dough helps it develop texture.

- Use as little flour as possible for dusting to keep dough from sticking to work surface.

- Fold dough toward you and push the dough down and away from you with the heels of your hands. Rotate dough one-fourth turn and repeat.

- Continue to knead until dough is smooth and elastic. The surface of the dough will look blistered.

- Don't think of kneading as a chore. Have fun with it—put on some favorite music and get into the rhythm. You'll be rewarded with the delicious aroma of freshly baked bread wafting all through the house.

Pizza Sauce

This recipe can be easily doubled and freezes well. For a chunky sauce, use the diced tomatoes. If you like a smoother sauce, opt for the crushed tomatoes.

½	cup beef or chicken broth
2	teaspoons dried basil
½	teaspoon dried oregano
1	tablespoon olive oil
¼	cup diced onion (about ½ small onion)
2	teaspoons minced garlic (about 4 medium cloves)
1	14½-oz. can diced or crushed tomatoes
3	ounces tomato paste (½ of a 6-oz. can)
½	teaspoon sugar
¼	teaspoon salt

◉ Heat broth on stove or in microwave just to a simmer. Remove from heat source, add basil and oregano, and steep 15 minutes.

◉ Heat oil in a large saucepan over medium-high heat. Add onion and cook 3–5 minutes, until tender. Add garlic and cook 1 minute more. Add broth with herbs along with the crushed tomatoes, tomato paste, sugar, and salt and bring to a boil. Reduce heat, cover, and simmer about 25–30 minutes, stirring occasionally.

Makes about 2 cups

Pizza Combos

Preheat oven to 450°F.

Start with a crust:
> Pizza Base Focaccia (pg. 89)
> French or other rustic bread, split lengthwise
> Whole pita breads
> Split English muffins

Place crust on baking sheet, add a sauce and any combination of toppings:

Pizza Sauce (pg. 90)
Shredded part-skim mozzarella cheese
Grated Parmesan cheese
Cooked Sweet Italian Sausage (pg. 117)
Sliced mushrooms
Sliced bell pepper
Thinly sliced onion
Black olives, pitted and halved

Barbecue Sauce (pg. 190)
Shredded 2% sharp Cheddar cheese
Cooked chicken breast strips
or steamed shrimp
Sliced bell pepper
Thinly sliced onion

Pesto (pg. 165)
Sliced aged Provolone cheese
Sliced Roma tomatoes
Sliced roasted red peppers
Chopped artichoke hearts

Fresh Tomato Salsa (pg. 27)
Shredded 2% Cheddar cheese
Cookied chicken breast strips
Canned black beans, rinsed and drained
Sliced green onions

Bake at 450°F as follows:
Focaccia: 12–15 minutes
French or rustic bread: 15–20 minutes
Whole pita bread: 12–15 minutes
Split English muffins: 10–12 minutes

Zucchini Bread

⅓	cup applesauce
2	large eggs
1½	cups shredded zucchini (about 2 small zucchinis)
1	teaspoon vanilla
2¼	teaspoons baking powder
½	teaspoon salt
½	teaspoon cinnamon
⅛	teaspoon ground nutmeg
½	cup dark brown sugar
¼	cup sugar
1¾	cups unbleached all-purpose flour
½	cup dried cranberries or raisins (optional)

◉ Preheat oven to 350°F. Coat loaf pan or 4 mini loaf pans with vegetable spray.

◉ In a large bowl combine applesauce, eggs, zucchini, and vanilla and stir well. Add baking powder, salt, cinnamon, and nutmeg and stir well. Add dark brown sugar and granulated sugar and stir well. Stir in flour just until combined—do not overmix. Fold in dried cranberries or raisins, if desired.

◉ Pour batter into prepared loaf pan(s). Bake for 1 hour to 1 hour and 10 minutes, until toothpick inserted in center comes out clean (bake mini loaf pans 30–40 minutes). Remove from pan(s) and cool on wire rack.

1 loaf or 4 mini loaves, about 12 servings

Aunti Bren's Banana Bread

Potassium-rich bananas help to restore lost body fluids and are a good source of soluble fiber. This bread is delicious warm, cold, or toasted. For an over-the-top breakfast, use this bread to make French toast topped with real maple syrup and sliced bananas.

⅓	cup applesauce
2	large eggs
3	very ripe bananas, mashed
1	teaspoon vanilla
1	teaspoon baking powder
½	teaspoon baking soda
½	teaspoon salt
½	teaspoon cinnamon
⅛	teaspoon ground nutmeg
½	cup dark brown sugar
1¾	cups unbleached all-purpose flour

◉ Preheat oven to 350°F. Coat loaf pan or mini loaf pans with vegetable spray.

◉ In a large bowl combine applesauce, eggs, bananas, and vanilla and stir well. Add baking powder, baking soda, salt, cinnamon, and nutmeg and stir well. Add brown sugar and stir well. Stir in flour just until combined—do not overmix.

◉ Pour batter into prepared pan(s). Bake for 45–55 minutes, until toothpick inserted in center comes out clean (bake mini loaves about 25–30 minutes). Remove from pan(s) and cool on wire rack.

1 loaf or 4 mini loaves, about 12 servings

Pumpkin Bread

⅓   cup applesauce

2   large eggs

1   15-oz. can solid-pack pumpkin (not pumpkin-pie mix)

1   teaspoon baking powder

½   teaspoon baking soda

½   teaspoon cinnamon

½   teaspoon ground ginger

½   teaspoon salt

¼   teaspoon ground nutmeg

½   cup dark brown sugar

1¾   cups unbleached all-purpose flour

½   cup dried cranberries or raisins (optional)

◉ Preheat oven to 350°F. Coat loaf pan or 4 mini loaf pans with vegetable spray.

◉ In a large bowl combine applesauce, eggs, and pumpkin and stir well. Add baking powder, baking soda, cinnamon, ginger, salt, and nutmeg and stir well. Add brown sugar and stir well. Stir in flour just until combined—do not overmix. Fold in dried cranberries or raisins, if desired.

◉ Pour into prepared pan(s). Bake about 1 hour, until toothpick inserted in center comes out clean (bake mini loaves 30–35 minutes). Remove from pan(s) and cool on wire rack.

Makes 1 loaf or 4 mini loaves, about 12 servings

Peanut Butter Bread

½   cup natural creamy-style peanut butter (no hydrogenated oils)

¼   cup sugar

¼   cup dark brown sugar

1   large egg

1   cup 2% milk or soy milk

2   teaspoons baking powder

1   teaspoon salt

2   cups unbleached all-purpose flour

◉ Preheat oven to 350°F. Coat loaf pan or mini loaf pans with vegetable spray.

◉ With an electric mixer, beat peanut butter, sugar, brown sugar, and egg until creamy. Add milk and beat to combine. Stir in baking powder and salt. Stir in flour just to combine—do not overmix.

◉ Pour into prepared pan(s). Bake 50 minutes to 1 hour, until toothpick inserted in center comes out clean (bake mini loaves 25–30 minutes). Remove from pan(s) and cool on wire rack.

1 loaf or 4 mini loaves, about 12 servings

Honey Butter

½   cup butter/canola oil blend, softened

¼   cup honey

◉ With an electric mixer, beat butter and honey together until combined and creamy, about 2 minutes. Spoon into a small jar or plastic container with lid. Refrigerate for up to 1 month.

Makes about ¾ cup

Blueberry Muffins

1	large egg
⅓	cup sugar
⅓	cup applesauce
¼	cup 2% milk or soy milk
2	tablespoons butter/canola blend, melted
1	teaspoon vanilla
2	cups unbleached all-purpose flour
1	tablespoon baking powder
½	teaspoon salt
1	cup fresh or frozen blueberries

◉ Preheat oven to 400°F. Line muffin pan with paper cups or coat with vegetable spray.

◉ In a medium bowl whisk together egg, sugar, applesauce, milk, butter, and vanilla. Add flour, baking powder, and salt and stir just to combine (batter will be lumpy). Fold in blueberries (if using frozen blueberries, do not thaw).

◉ Fill muffin cups three-fourths full. Bake about 20 minutes, until toothpick inserted in center comes out clean. Remove from pan immediately and cool on wire rack.

Variations

Oatmeal Raisin Muffins: Omit blueberries. Substitute 1 cup oatmeal for 1 cup of the flour. Add ½ teaspoon cinnamon and ⅛ teaspoon ground nutmeg with the salt. Fold in 1 cup raisins.

Cranberry Lemon Muffins: Omit blueberries. Add 1 teaspoon lemon zest (grated rind) with the vanilla. Fold in 1 cup fresh cranberries (coarsely chopped) or dried cranberries.

Makes 1 dozen muffins

Weekend Roast Beef

Serve this roast with Garlic Mashed Potatoes (pg. 168) and Pan Gravy (pg. 134), if desired. Slice leftover roast beef thinly and place on toasted hoagie rolls. Top with aged Provolone cheese and broil 2–3 minutes to make Philly-style sandwiches.

1	4-pound round or rump roast, trimmed
1	tablespoon olive or canola oil
1	tablespoon Worcestershire sauce
1	teaspoon salt
1	teaspoon onion powder
½	teaspoon garlic powder
½	teaspoon dried thyme
½	teaspoon black pepper

◉ Heat oven to 425°F. Place roast in shallow roasting pan. Drizzle with oil and Worcestershire sauce. Sprinkle with seasonings. Roast for 20 minutes. Reduce oven temperature to 325°F. Roast until internal temperature reaches 140°F (medium rare), about 1½ hours.

◉ Transfer to serving platter and allow roast to rest for 15 minutes before slicing. Prepare Pan Gravy (pg. 134), if desired.

Makes 8–10 servings

Home-Style Pot Roast with Root Vegetables

2	tablespoons olive oil
1	3½- to 4-pound chuck or round roast, trimmed
1	teaspoon salt
½	teaspoon black pepper
2	bay leaves
1	tablespoon Worcestershire sauce
1	14½-oz. can beef broth
1	cup thinly sliced onion (about 1 medium onion)
8	medium carrots, cut into 2-inch pieces
3	medium onions, quartered
6	medium potatoes, peeled and quartered (all-purpose, russet, or Yukon Gold)
3	ribs celery, cut into 2-inch pieces

◉ Heat oil in a Dutch oven over medium-high heat. Add roast and brown on all sides.

◉ Add salt, pepper, bay leaves, Worcestershire sauce, beef broth, and enough cold water to almost cover roast. Scatter sliced onion around roast. Bring to a boil, cover, reduce heat and simmer about 2½ hours.

◉ Add carrots, onions, potatoes, and celery and bring back to a boil. Reduce heat, cover, and simmer about 45 minutes to 1 hour, until roast and vegetables are fork-tender. Remove roast and vegetables to serving platter and prepare gravy.

(continued on next page)

Pot Roast Gravy

◉ Skim any excess fat from broth and add enough water to equal about 2 cups. Bring to a boil. Shake together ½ cup cold water and ¼ cup all-purpose flour in a lidded jar until well blended. Whisk the flour slurry into the broth in a slow, steady stream. Continue to whisk for 1–2 minutes until thick and of even consistency. Taste and season with salt and pepper, if desired.

Makes 8 servings

Herbes de Provence

1	tablespoon dried rosemary
1	tablespoon dried thyme
1	tablespoon dried savory
1	tablespoon dried lavender flowers
1	teaspoon dried marjoram
1	teaspoon dried basil

◉ Mix ingredients together and store in an airtight container.

Makes ¼ cup

Horseradish Pot Roast

2	tablespoons olive oil
1	3½- to 4-pound chuck or round roast, trimmed
1	teaspoon salt
½	teaspoon black pepper
3	ounces prepared horseradish (about ½ of a 6-oz. jar)
1	14½-oz. can beef broth
8	medium carrots, cut into 2-inch pieces
2	medium onions, quartered
6	medium potatoes, peeled and quartered (all-purpose, russet, or Yukon Gold)

◉ Heat oil in a Dutch oven over medium-high heat. Add roast and brown on all sides. Season with salt and pepper. Spread horseradish on top of roast. Add beef broth and enough water to almost cover roast. Bring to a boil, cover, reduce heat and simmer 2½ hours.

◉ Add carrots, onions, and potatoes and bring back to a boil. Cover, reduce heat, and simmer 45 minutes to 1 hour, until roast and vegetables are fork-tender.

◉ Remove roast and vegetables to serving platter. Prepare and serve with Pot Roast Gravy (pg. 99), if desired.

Makes 8 servings

Old-Fashioned Beef Stew

1	tablespoon olive oil
1	1- to 1½-pound chuck, round, or sirloin roast, trimmed and cut into 2-inch cubes
2	cups diced onion (about 1 large onion)
2	14½-oz. cans beef broth
1	tablespoon Worcestershire sauce
2	bay leaves
½	teaspoon herbes de Provence
½	teaspoon salt
¼	teaspoon black pepper
2	large all-purpose potatoes, peeled and cubed
3	medium carrots, cut into 1-inch pieces
2	ribs celery, sliced
1	cup frozen peas
¼	cup cold water
2	tablespoons all-purpose flour

◉ Heat oil in a Dutch oven over medium-high heat. Add beef cubes and brown on all sides. Add onion and cook about 5 minutes, until onion is translucent.

◉ Add broth, Worcestershire sauce, bay leaves, herbes de Provence, salt, and pepper. Bring to a boil. Reduce heat, cover, and simmer about 1½ hours, until beef is almost tender.

◉ Add potatoes, carrots, and celery and return to a boil. Reduce heat, cover, and simmer 30 minutes, until beef and vegetables are tender. Add peas and cook 2–3 minutes more.

◉ Shake water and flour together in a lidded jar until well blended. Whisk flour slurry into stew in a slow, steady stream until thick and bubbly. Simmer 2 more minutes, stirring occasionally. Serve with a crusty bread to dip in the gravy.

Makes 5–6 servings

Beef Stroganoff

1½	tablespoons olive oil
1	2-pound sirloin roast, trimmed and cut into 1½-inch cubes
1	cup thinly sliced onion (about 1 medium onion)
1	cup beef broth
2	tablespoons tomato paste
1	teaspoon Worcestershire sauce
½	teaspoon minced garlic (about 1 medium clove)
½	teaspoon salt
¼	teaspoon black pepper
8	ounces fresh white mushrooms, stems removed and caps sliced
1	cup reduced-fat sour cream or plain yogurt
	Hot egg noodles

◉ Heat oil in a Dutch oven over medium-high heat. Add beef cubes and brown an all sides. Transfer beef to platter and set aside.

◉ Add onion and cook about 5 minutes, until translucent. Add broth, tomato paste, Worcestershire sauce, garlic, salt, and pepper and stir to combine. Return beef to Dutch oven, stir into sauce and bring to a boil. Reduce heat, cover, and simmer about 1½ hours, until beef is fork-tender.

◉ Uncover, add mushrooms, and simmer 5–7 minutes, until mushrooms are tender. While still at a simmer, stir in sour cream or yogurt and heat through, about 1–2 minutes (do not boil). Serve stroganoff over hot egg noodles.

Makes 8 servings

Beef Cabernet

Paired with a simple salad and a loaf of crusty bread, this main attraction is elegant enough for a small dinner party and hearty enough for Sunday dinner with the family.

3	slices center-cut bacon
1	tablespoon olive oil
1	2-pound sirloin roast, trimmed and cut into 1½- to 2-inch cubes
1	teaspoon minced garlic (about 2 medium cloves)
1	cup beef broth
1	cup Cabernet Sauvignon
2	tablespoons tomato paste
½	teaspoon dried thyme
½	teaspoon herbes de Provence
½	teaspoon salt
¼	teaspoon black pepper
2	bay leaves
4	medium carrots, cut into 1-inch pieces
15–18	pearl onions, peeled
8	ounces fresh white mushrooms, stems removed
	Hot rice, egg noodles, or mashed potatoes

◉ In a Dutch oven cook bacon over medium-high heat until crisp. Remove bacon, drain on paper towels, and set aside.

◉ Add oil and beef cubes and brown an all sides. Add garlic, broth, wine, tomato paste, thyme, herbes de Provence, salt, pepper, and bay leaves and bring to a boil. Reduce heat, cover and simmer about 1 hour and 15 minutes—beef should be almost fork-tender.

◉ Add carrots, onions, and mushrooms and bring back to a boil. Reduce heat, cover, and simmer 30–40 minutes, until vegetables and beef are tender.

◉ Serve over hot rice, egg noodles, or mashed potatoes and top with crumbled bacon.

Makes 6 servings

Sirloin Tips on Rice

This is my husband's absolute favorite—he never tires of it!

1½	tablespoons olive oil
1	2-pound sirloin roast, trimmed and cut into 2-inch cubes
2	large onions, sliced thin
1	cup beef broth
1	tablespoon Worcestershire sauce
½	teaspoon salt
½	teaspoon black pepper
	Hot jasmine, basmati, or white rice

◉ Heat oil in a Dutch oven over medium-high heat. Add beef cubes and brown on all sides. Add onions and cook about 5 minutes.

◉ Add broth, Worcestershire sauce, salt, and pepper and bring to a boil. Reduce heat, cover, and simmer about 1 hour and 30 minutes to 1 hour and 45 minutes, stirring occasionally, until beef is fork-tender and the liquid has reduced to a thin sauce.

◉ Serve over hot jasmine, basmati, or white rice.

Note: for a thicker, gravy-like sauce, in a lidded jar, shake together ¼ cup cold water and 2 tablespoons flour until blended. Whisk flour slurry into beef tips about 1 tablespoon at a time until you reach desired consistency and simmer 1–2 minutes.

Makes 6 servings

Hungarian Goulash

1½   tablespoons olive oil

1   2-pound sirloin roast, trimmed and cut into 1½-inch cubes

2   cups thinly sliced onion (about 1 large onion)

1   cup thinly sliced green bell pepper (about 1 medium pepper)

1   teaspoon minced garlic (about 2 medium cloves)

1   14½-oz. can diced tomatoes

1   14½-oz. can beef broth

1   tablespoon paprika

1   teaspoon salt

¼   teaspoon black pepper

     Hot egg noodles

◉ Heat oil in a Dutch oven over medium-high heat. Add beef cubes and brown on all sides. Add onion and bell pepper and cook about 5 minutes.

◉ Add garlic and cook 1 minute. Add tomatoes, broth, paprika, salt, and pepper, stir well to combine, and bring to a boil. Reduce heat, cover, and simmer about 2 hours, stirring occasionally, until beef is fork-tender.

◉ Serve over hot egg noodles.

Makes 6 servings

Pepper Steak

1	tablespoon olive or canola oil
1	pound boneless beef round or sirloin steak, cut across the grain into thin strips*
1	cup thinly sliced onion (about 1 medium)
1	cup beef broth
2	tablespoons lite soy sauce
1	tablespoon Worcestershire sauce
½	teaspoon ground ginger
¼	teaspoon salt
¼	teaspoon black pepper
1	cup thinly sliced green bell pepper (about 1 medium pepper)
1	cup thinly sliced red bell pepper (about 1 medium pepper)
	Hot jasmine or white rice

◉ Heat oil in a skillet over medium-high heat. Add beef strips and cook about 2 minutes—turning once—to slightly brown. Add onion slices and cook about 5 minutes.

◉ Add broth, soy sauce, Worcestershire sauce, ginger, salt, and pepper and bring to a boil. Reduce heat, cover, and simmer 45 minutes.

◉ Add green and red bell pepper, cover, and simmer another 15–20 minutes, until peppers and beef are fork-tender. Serve over hot rice.

Place beef in freezer for 30 minutes for easier slicing.

Makes 4 servings

Mom's Onion Swiss Steak

This is my mom's version of Swiss Steak with a few additions of my own to give it more beef flavor. She always served it with plenty of mashed potatoes and whatever vegetable was on hand. There were never any leftovers!

1¼	pounds cubed steak
½	cup all-purpose flour
¼	teaspoon salt
¼	teaspoon black pepper
¼	teaspoon garlic powder
¼	teaspoon Old Bay seasoning
1½	tablespoons canola or olive oil
2	cups thinly sliced onion (about 1 large onion)
1	cup beef broth
1	teaspoon Worcestershire sauce
¼	cup cold water
2	tablespoons all-purpose flour

◉ Cut steak into 8–10 equal pieces. Mix flour, salt, pepper, garlic powder, and Old Bay seasoning in a shallow bowl or glass pie pan.

◉ Heat oil in a large skillet over medium heat. Dredge steaks in flour mixture, add to skillet and brown, about 5 minutes on each side. Remove steaks from skillet and set aside.

◉ Add onion to skillet and cook about 5–7 minutes, until translucent. Stir in broth and Worcestershire sauce. Return steaks to skillet and bring to a boil. Reduce heat, cover, and simmer about 1 hour, until beef is fork-tender. Remove steaks from skillet and set aside.

◉ In a lidded jar, shake together water and flour until well blended. Whisk flour slurry into pan drippings in skillet, 1 tablespoon at a time, until desired consistency. Return steaks to skillet and simmer 2 minutes.

Makes 4–5 servings

Shepherd's Pie

The basics of this recipe came from my friend Judy Colwell nearly twenty years ago. Although I've altered it slightly, it still evokes a sense of warmth and home for me.

1	recipe Basic Mashed Potatoes (pg. 168)*
1½	pounds lean hamburger
½	cup diced onion (about 1 small)
½	cup diced green bell pepper (about ½ medium)
½	cup diced celery (about 1 rib)
2	teaspoons Worcestershire sauce
¼	teaspoon salt
⅛	teaspoon black pepper
1	10¾-oz. can condensed tomato soup
8	ounces frozen peas or green beans, thawed
1½	cups shredded 2% sharp Cheddar cheese (about 6 oz)**

◉ Prepare mashed potatoes.

◉ In the meantime, cook hamburger, onion, bell pepper, and celery in a skillet over medium heat until beef is browned and vegetables are tender, about 10 minutes.

◉ Preheat oven to 350°F. Add Worcestershire sauce, salt, black pepper, and tomato soup and heat through. Spoon beef mixture into a 2-quart casserole dish. Top with peas or green beans. Spoon mashed potatoes in mounds atop the vegetables. Sprinkle Cheddar cheese atop the potato mounds. Bake about 25–30 minutes, until bubbly and cheese is golden. Allow to rest 15 minutes before serving.

To save time, use leftover mashed potatoes if you have them. You'll need about 3–4 cups.
**To lower the lactose, use full-fat sharp Cheddar cheese instead of the 2%.*

Makes 6 servings

Jean's Hamburger and Rice

One evening I asked my husband what was one of his favorite dishes that his mom used to make. His immediate reply was Hamburger and Rice. I had never heard of it, so I asked him to get the recipe from her. He called his mom and wrote it down on a Post-it note (which I still have taped to my refrigerator 5 years later). I have altered it only slightly.

1	pound lean hamburger
1	cup diced onion (about 1 medium onion)
½	cup diced green bell pepper (about ½ medium pepper)
1	cup sliced celery (about 2 ribs)
4	ounces fresh white or baby bella (cremini) mushrooms, stems removed and sliced
¼	teaspoon salt
⅛	teaspoon black pepper
3	cups beef broth
1	tablespoon Worcestershire sauce
1	cup white or jasmine rice

◉ In a large skillet cook the hamburger, onion, bell pepper, celery, and mushrooms over medium heat until meat is browned and vegetables are tender, about 10 minutes.

◉ Add remaining ingredients, stirring well to combine, and bring to a boil. Cover, reduce heat, and simmer about 20 minutes, until rice is tender and most of the broth has been absorbed.

Makes 4 servings

Þren's Meatloaf

Using a large baking dish, rather than a loaf pan, allows the meatloaf to develop a crispy crust on the sides as well as the top. Don't forget the mashed potatoes!

1½	pounds lean hamburger
½	cup diced onion (about 1 small onion)
½	cup diced green bell pepper (about ½ medium pepper)
12	low-fat butter-type crackers, crushed
¼	cup plain bread crumbs
¼	cup ketchup
2	teaspoons Worcestershire sauce
1	large egg
½	teaspoon herbes de Provence or Italian seasoning
¼	teaspoon salt
¼	teaspoon black pepper

◉ Heat oven to 375°F. Combine all ingredients in a large bowl and mix with hands until just combined. Place in a 13 x 9 baking dish and shape into a 10 x 6-inch loaf.

◉ Bake about 1 hour to 1 hour and 10 minutes, until no longer pink in center. Let rest 10–15 minutes for ease in slicing.

Variation
Mini Meatloaves: Spray muffin pan with vegetable spray. Spoon beef mixture evenly into 12 muffin cups. Bake for 25–30 minutes or until no longer pink in center. Let rest 5 minutes before serving. Allow 2 mini meatloaves per person.

Makes 6 servings

Venison Steak with Peppers and Onions

1	tablespoon butter/canola oil blend
1	tablespoon olive oil
1½	pounds venison loin steak, sliced very thin*
2	cups thinly sliced onion (about 1 large onion)
1	cup thinly sliced green bell pepper (about 1 medium pepper)
½	teaspoon salt
¼	teaspoon black pepper
¼	teaspoon garlic powder

◉ Heat butter and olive oil over medium-high heat in a large skillet. Add venison and cook about 5 minutes, stirring occasionally, until browned. Add remaining ingredients and stir well. Reduce heat to medium. Cover and cook until meat is tender, about 25–30 minutes.

Note: Place meat in freezer for 30 minutes for easier slicing.

Makes 6 servings

Hunter's Stew

1	tablespoon olive oil
1½	pounds venison loin or stew meat, trimmed and cut into 1½-inch cubes
2	14½-oz. cans beef broth
1	tablespoon Worcestershire sauce
2	bay leaves
½	teaspoon salt
¼	teaspoon black pepper
2	cups peeled and cubed all-purpose potatoes (about 2 medium potatoes)
2	cups peeled and cubed sweet potatoes (about 2 medium sweet potatoes)
4	medium carrots, cut into 1-inch pieces (about 2 cups)
1	cup diced onion (about 1 medium onion)
1	cup sliced celery (about 2 ribs)
¼	cup cold water
2	tablespoons all-purpose flour

- Heat oil in a Dutch oven over medium-high heat. Add venison cubes and brown on all sides. Add broth, Worcestershire sauce, bay leaves, salt, and pepper and bring to a boil.

- Reduce heat, cover, and simmer about 1½ hours, until venison is almost tender.

- Add both potatoes, carrots, onion, and celery and bring to a boil. Reduce heat, cover, and simmer about 30 minutes, until venison and vegetables are tender.

- Shake water and flour together in a lidded jar. Whisk flour slurry into stew in a slow, steady stream. Simmer another 2 minutes, until thick and bubbly.

Makes 5–6 servings

Easy Pork Tenderloin

1	pound pork tenderloin
1	tablespoon olive oil
1	teaspoon herbes de Provence
½	teaspoon garlic powder
¼	teaspoon salt
¼	teaspoon black pepper

◉ Heat oven to 425°F. Place tenderloin in a shallow roasting pan. Drizzle with olive oil and sprinkle with seasonings. Roast for 25–30 minutes until meat thermometer registers 155–160°F. Allow to rest 10 minutes before slicing.

Variations

Apricot-Glazed Pork Tenderloin: Omit olive oil and seasonings. Combine ½ cup apricot preserves, 2 teaspoons lite soy sauce, and ⅛ teaspoon ground ginger. Drizzle apricot glaze on pork loin and roast as directed.

Maple-Dijon Pork Tenderloin: Omit olive oil and seasonings. Combine ¼ cup pure maple syrup, 1 tablespoon Dijon mustard, ½ teaspoon dried thyme, ¼ teaspoon salt, and ¼ teaspoon black pepper. Drizzle syrup mixture over tenderloin and roast as directed.

Makes 4 servings

Herbed Pork Loin with Roasted Vegetables

1	2- to 2½-pound boneless pork loin roast, trimmed
6	medium carrots, cut into 1-inch pieces
2	small onions, quartered
6	medium potatoes (all-purpose, red, or Yukon Gold), unpeeled, washed, and quartered
1½	tablespoons olive oil
1	teaspoon dried sage
½	teaspoon dried thyme
½	teaspoon dried rosemary
½	teaspoon salt
¼	teaspoon black pepper
	Cranberry-Horseradish Sauce (pg. 193)

◉ Heat oven to 375°F. Place pork loin in roasting pan and surround it with carrots, onions, and potatoes. Drizzle roast and vegetables with olive oil and sprinkle with seasonings. Roast for 30 minutes per pound—about 1 hour to 1 hour and 15 minutes—until meat thermometer registers 160°F.

◉ Let roast rest 10–15 minutes before slicing. Serve with Cranberry Horseradish Sauce, if desired.

Variations
Curried Pork Loin with Roasted Vegetables: Substitute 3 large sweet potatoes, peeled and cut into 1-inch slices, for the all-purpose potatoes. Omit sage, thyme, and rosemary. Sprinkle roast and vegetables with 2 teaspoons Curry Blend (pg. 115) or curry powder. Serve with Mango Chutney (pg. 192), if desired.

Italian Pork Loin with Roasted Vegetables: Substitute 3 medium bell peppers (green, yellow, or red), seeded and cut into quarters, for the carrots. Substitute red onions for the white onions. Omit sage, thyme and rosemary. Sprinkle roast and vegetables with 1 tablespoon fennel seeds, 1 teaspoon Italian seasoning, and ½ teaspoon garlic powder.

Makes 6–8 servings

Curry Blend

4	teaspoons coriander
2	teaspoons cumin
2	teaspoons paprika
2	teaspoons turmeric
1	teaspoon cayenne pepper
½	teaspoon ground cloves
½	teaspoon ground cardamom

◉ Mix all ingredients together and store in an airtight container.

Makes ¼ cup

Homemade Sausage

Sausage was on my don't-even-think-about-it list for a long time. Whether it is the preservatives used or the high saturated fat content (or both), store-bought sausage always sends me straight to the bathroom. Then it hit me: if I made my own sausage, I could control the fat content, and there would be no need for preservatives.

I purchased a meat grinder for $25 at True Value Hardware and was in business! If you're not familiar with this device, it's a simple-to-use, manual meat and vegetable grinder made of cast iron. It was a staple piece of equipment in home kitchens before the food processor became popular—your mother and/or grandmother probably had one. The texture of the ground meat from a grinder is far superior to that of a food processor, and for that reason alone it is worth the small investment. Properly cared for, a meat grinder will last a lifetime. If grinding your own meat seems like too much of a chore, that's okay—hand the meat to your butcher and ask him or her to trim the fat and grind it for you.

Purchasing whole boneless pork loins (about 3–4 pounds each) when they go on sale (often half price) makes it very economical to make your own sausage. Unless you have a kitchen scale, note the weight on the package before you begin as this will help you to estimate the volume of the final ground meat. Trim most of the fat from the pork loin—this will account for approximately 1/4–1/2 pound. Cut into large chunks and grind. With 1 pork loin, you can make all three of the following sausages or prepare just one and triple the seasonings. Once you've tried making homemade sausage, you can always vary the seasonings to suit your family's taste. You can also substitute turkey or chicken breast meat for the pork loin.

Homemade Sausage

Farmer's Sausage

1–1¼ pounds ground pork loin

1	tablespoon dried sage
1	teaspoon dried parsley
½	teaspoon dried thyme
½	teaspoon dried basil
½	teaspoon marjoram
½	teaspoon chili powder
½	teaspoon garlic powder
½	teaspoon salt
½	teaspoon black pepper

Sweet Italian Sausage

1–1¼ pounds ground pork loin

1	tablespoon fennel seeds
½	tablespoon Italian seasoning
1	teaspoon black pepper
½	teaspoon salt

Breakfast Sausage

1–1¼ pounds ground pork loin

2	teaspoons dried sage
½	teaspoon salt
½	teaspoon summer savory
½	teaspoon marjoram
½	teaspoon black pepper

◉ Combine ingredients from sausage of choice above and mix well. Cover and chill at least 2 hours. If not cooking immediately after chilling, wrap in plastic wrap in ½–1¼ pound bulk packages or shape into patties. Place in a ziplock bag and freeze.

◉ Because it is so lean, you will need to add a little olive oil to your skillet when cooking the sausage. Cook over medium heat until browned, about 5–10 minutes. Drain on paper towels.

Sausage Bread

1	loaf frozen white bread dough, thawed to package directions
¼	pound sliced aged Provolone cheese
½	pound Sweet Italian Sausage (pg. 117), cooked and drained on paper towels
¼	cup grated Parmesan cheese
	Cornmeal for dusting
	Marinara Sauce (pg. 163)

◉ Roll out bread dough on a floured surface into a rectangle about 12 x 8 inches. Layer Provolone slices down the center of the dough. Top Provolone with cooked sausage and sprinkle with grated Parmesan. Fold one side over center lengthwise. Repeat with other side and pinch to seal. Fold over ends and pinch to seal.

◉ Coat a baking sheet with vegetable spray and dust with cornmeal. Place loaf on prepared baking sheet seam-side down. Cover with plastic wrap or clean kitchen towel and let rise 30 minutes.

◉ Preheat oven to 400°F. Bake 25–30 minutes, until golden. Serve with homemade or bottled marinara sauce for dipping, if desired.

6 servings, 2 slices each

Herb Roasted Chicken and Vegetables

This easy-to-prepare dish takes care of itself in the oven. That means you have time for the more important things in life—like helping the kids with their homework or enjoying a glass of wine and some conversation with a friend.

1	4- to 5-pound roasting chicken
3	medium onions, quartered
6	medium carrots, cut into 2-inch pieces
3	ribs celery, cut into 2-inch pieces
6	medium all-purpose potatoes, washed and quartered
2	tablespoons olive oil
1	teaspoon poultry seasoning
1	teaspoon Italian seasoning
½	teaspoon paprika
½	teaspoon salt
¼	teaspoon black pepper

◉ Heat oven to 375°F. Remove gizzards from chicken and discard. Rinse chicken under cold water and pat dry with paper towels. Place chicken in roasting pan. Arrange onions, carrots, celery, and potatoes around chicken in pan. Drizzle chicken and vegetables with olive oil and sprinkle with seasonings.

◉ Roast for 20 minutes per pound of chicken—about 1 hour and 15 minutes to 1 hour and 45 minutes. Chicken is done when leg pulls easily from body and juices run clear when thickest part of chicken is pierced with a fork. Allow chicken to rest 10 minutes before carving.

Variation
Tarragon Roast Chicken and Vegetables: Omit poultry seasoning, Italian seasoning, and paprika. Add 2 teaspoons dried tarragon.

Makes 6 servings

Chicken Cacciatore

1	tablespoon olive oil
8	boneless, skinless chicken thighs
1	cup diced onion (about 1 medium onion)
1	teaspoon minced garlic (about 2 medium cloves)
8	ounces fresh white mushrooms, stems removed and caps sliced
1	14½-oz. can diced tomatoes
4	tablespoons tomato paste
1	teaspoon Italian seasoning
½	teaspoon salt
¼	teaspoon black pepper
	Hot spaghetti or fettuccini
1	tablespoon fresh basil, torn or chopped

◉ Heat olive oil in a large skillet over medium-high heat. Add chicken thighs and brown, about 4–5 minutes on each side. Remove thighs and set aside. Add onion and cook about 5 minutes, until translucent. Add garlic and mushrooms and cook another 5 minutes, until mushrooms are tender.

◉ Return chicken to skillet. Add tomatoes, tomato paste, Italian seasoning, salt, and pepper; stir to combine and bring to a boil. Reduce heat, cover, and simmer 25–30 minutes, until chicken is very tender.

◉ Serve over hot spaghetti or fettuccini and garnish with fresh basil.

Makes 4 servings

Chicken Paprika

1	tablespoon canola or olive oil
8	boneless, skinless chicken thighs
1	cup thinly sliced onion (about 1 medium onion)
1	teaspoon minced garlic (about 2 medium cloves)
1	8-oz. can tomato sauce (about 1 cup)
1	cup chicken broth
1	tablespoon paprika
½	teaspoon salt
¼	teaspoon black pepper
1	cup reduced-fat sour cream or plain yogurt
	Hot egg noodles

◉ Heat oil in a large skillet over medium-high heat. Add chicken thighs and brown, about 4–5 minutes on each side. Remove thighs and set aside.

◉ Add onion and cook about 5 minutes, until translucent. Add garlic and cook 1 minute.

◉ Return chicken to skillet and add tomato sauce, broth, paprika, salt, and pepper and bring to a boil. Reduce heat, cover, and simmer about 25–30 minutes, until chicken is very tender and sauce has reduced. Stir in sour cream or yogurt and heat through—do not boil.

◉ Serve over hot egg noodles.

Makes 4 servings

Chicken Parmesan

If you are lactose intolerant, omit the mozzarella from this recipe and garnish with extra Parmesan if you wish—it will be just as delicious! Serve with a side of hot spaghetti or fettuccini, extra sauce, and rustic bread for a satisfying meal.

½	cup plain bread crumbs
4	tablespoons grated Parmesan cheese, divided
1	teaspoon Italian seasoning
¼	teaspoon salt
¼	teaspoon black pepper
1	large egg
1½	tablespoons olive oil
4	boneless, skinless chicken breast halves (about 1 pound)
1½	cups Marinara Sauce (pg. 163) or bottled sauce
1	cup shredded part-skim mozzarella cheese

- In a shallow bowl combine bread crumbs, 2 tablespoons Parmesan cheese, Italian seasoning, salt, and pepper. In another shallow bowl lightly beat the egg.
- Heat olive oil in a large skillet over medium heat. Dip chicken breast halves in beaten egg, dredge in bread crumb mixture, and place in skillet. Cook until browned and no longer pink inside, about 5–6 minutes on each side. Add Marinara Sauce and heat through. Sprinkle with mozzarella, reduce heat, cover and cook another 3–5 minutes, until cheese has melted. Garnish with remaining 2 tablespoons Parmesan.

Variation
Turkey Parmesan: Substitute turkey cutlets for the chicken breasts.

Makes 4 servings

Paella

1	tablespoon olive oil
1	pound boneless, skinless chicken breast, cut into 1-inch strips
1	cup diced onion (about 1 medium onion)
1	cup thinly sliced red bell pepper (about 1 medium pepper)
1	teaspoon minced garlic (about 2 medium cloves)
1	14½-oz. can diced tomatoes
1	14½-oz. can chicken broth
1	teaspoon salt
½	teaspoon black pepper
¼	teaspoon ground cumin
	Pinch of saffron (optional)
2	cups jasmine rice
8	ounces medium shrimp, peeled and deveined
12	Littleneck clams, scrubbed
1	cup frozen peas

◉ Heat olive oil in a Dutch oven over medium-high heat. Add chicken and cook about 7 minutes, until golden brown. Remove chicken and set aside.

◉ Add onion and bell pepper and cook about 5 minutes, until onion is translucent. Add garlic and cook 1 minute. Stir in tomatoes and cook 5 minutes. Add broth, salt, pepper, cumin, and saffron, if desired, and bring to a boil. Add rice and return chicken to the pot.

◉ Reduce heat, cover, and simmer 20 minutes. Add shrimp, clams, and peas. Cover and simmer 5 minutes. Remove from heat and let stand, covered, another 5 minutes before serving.

Makes 6 servings

Chicken Pot Pie

1	recipe Basic Mashed Potatoes (pg. 168) or 1-crust Standard Pastry Dough (pg. 197)
1	tablespoon olive oil
1	cup diced onion (about 1 medium onion)
1	cup sliced celery (about 2 ribs)
½	cup diced green bell pepper (about ½ medium pepper)
1½	cups chicken broth
1	cup 2% milk or ½ cup soy milk & ½ cup water
4	tablespoons all-purpose flour
½	teaspoon poultry seasoning
½	teaspoon salt
¼	teaspoon black pepper
2½–3	cups cooked chicken, chopped
1	cup frozen peas

◉ Prepare Mashed Potatoes (you can use leftover mashed potatoes if you wish) or Standard Pastry Dough and set aside.

◉ Heat olive oil in a Dutch oven over medium heat. Add onion, celery, and bell pepper and cook until tender, about 5–7 minutes. Add chicken broth and bring to a boil.

◉ Shake together milk and flour in a lidded jar until well blended. Whisk milk and flour slurry into chicken broth in a slow, steady stream until thick and bubbly. Add poultry seasoning, salt, pepper, chicken, and peas and stir to combine.

◉ Heat oven to 400°F. Coat a 2-quart rectangular casserole dish with vegetable spray. Spoon chicken mixture into casserole.

• **For potato topping:** Top casserole with potatoes, spreading evenly to the edges of the casserole dish.

◉ **For pastry topping:** On a lightly floured surface, roll dough into 12 x 8-inch rectangle, fold into quarters and cut slits in pastry. Place on top of casserole, unfold and flute edges to casserole dish to seal.

◉ Bake for 30–35 minutes. Let stand 15–20 minutes before serving.

Makes 6 servings

Curried Chicken

This earthy dish is best served over hot rice with warm tortillas on the side. Traditionally it is served with condiments such as chopped green onions, raisins, and mango chutney. You can substitute 1½ tablespoons Curry Blend (pg. 115) for the five-spice blend below.

1½	pounds boneless, skinless chicken breasts
2	14½-oz. cans chicken broth, divided
2	bay leaves
½	teaspoon minced garlic (about 1 medium clove)
½	teaspoon salt
1½	tablespoons butter/canola oil blend
1	cup diced onion (about 1 medium onion)
½	cup diced celery (about 1 rib)
1	apple, peeled, cored, and diced (about 1 medium apple)

Five-spice blend:

1	tablespoon curry powder
½	teaspoon ground cumin
½	teaspoon chili powder
¼	teaspoon ground ginger
¼	teaspoon turmeric
2	tablespoons all-purpose flour

◉ In a large skillet place chicken, 1 can of broth, bay leaves, garlic, and salt and bring to a boil. Reduce heat, cover, and simmer about 20–30 minutes, until chicken is no longer pink inside. (Time will depend on thickness of chicken breasts.) Remove chicken from broth and set aside until cool enough to handle.

◉ In the meantime, melt butter in a Dutch oven over medium heat. Add onion, celery, and apple and cook 10–12 minutes, until very tender. Add 1 cup broth and five-spice blend and cook another 5 minutes. Shake together ¾ cup broth and flour in a lidded jar.

◉ Whisk broth and flour slurry into Dutch oven in a slow, steady stream and cook about 2 minutes, until thickened.

◉ Shred chicken, return to pot, and simmer about 5 minutes to heat through.

Makes 6 servings

Poached Chicken

This gentle cooking method produces a very moist and tender chicken breast. Serve warm with a sauce such as Velouté (pg. 164) or cool and use for chicken salad.

4	boneless, skinless chicken breast halves
1	cup chicken broth
½	cup diced onion (about 1 small onion)
½	cup diced carrot (about 1 medium carrot)
1	bay leaf
½	teaspoon rubbed sage
¼	teaspoon salt
⅛	teaspoon black pepper

◉ Place all ingredients in a large skillet and bring to a boil. Reduce heat to barely simmering—do not cover. Barely simmer for 20–30 minutes, basting occasionally, until chicken is no longer pink inside. (Time will depend on thickness of chicken breasts.)

Makes 4 servings

Chicken Tenders

Chicken tenders were made for dipping in a creamy sauce. Some suggestions are: Buttermilk Herb Dressing (pg. 66), Honey-Dijon Dressing (pg. 67), and Roasted Red Pepper Dipping Sauce (pg. 191).

1½	pounds boneless, skinless chicken breasts
½	cup all-purpose flour
½	cup plain bread crumbs
2	teaspoons Old Bay seasoning
1	teaspoon garlic powder
½	teaspoon salt
¼	teaspoon black pepper
1	large egg
½	cup skim, 2%, or soy milk

- Heat oven to 400°F. Cut each chicken breast into 1-inch strips.

- In a shallow bowl combine the flour, bread crumbs, Old Bay seasoning, garlic powder, salt, and pepper.

- In a second shallow bowl whisk together egg and milk.

- Coat a baking sheet with vegetable spray. Dip chicken strips in egg wash, dredge in flour mixture, and place on prepared baking sheet. Lightly coat top of chicken with vegetable spray. Bake about 20 minutes, until golden brown and no longer pink inside.

Makes 6 servings

Swiss Chicken Casserole

1	cup chicken broth
4	ounces fresh white or cremini mushrooms, stems removed and caps sliced
½	cup diced onion (about 1 small onion)
1	cup diced celery (about 2 ribs)
½	cup diced green bell pepper (about ½ medium pepper)
2	tablespoons butter/canola blend
2	tablespoons all-purpose flour
1½	cups skim milk or ¾ cup soy milk & ¾ cup water
½	teaspoon salt
¼	teaspoon black pepper
2	cups cooked white or jasmine rice
2	cups chopped cooked chicken
1	cup shredded Swiss cheese

◉ Preheat oven to 350°F. Heat broth in a medium saucepan to boiling. Add mushrooms, onion, celery, and bell pepper. Reduce heat, cover, and simmer 5 minutes. Remove from heat and set aside.

◉ In a large skillet melt butter over medium heat. Whisk in flour and cook 1 minute, whisking constantly. Whisk in milk in a slow, steady stream. Cook 2–3 minutes, until thick and creamy. Season with salt and pepper. Stir in vegetables with broth. Add rice and chicken and stir to combine.

◉ Spoon into a 2-quart casserole dish and bake for 25 minutes. Sprinkle cheese on top of casserole and bake another 5–10 minutes, until cheese has melted. Allow to stand for 10 minutes before serving.

Makes 6 servings

Garlic and Lemon Cornish Game Hens

2	1½-pound Cornish game hens
1	large head of garlic
1	tablespoon olive oil
3	tablespoons fresh lemon juice (about 1 medium lemon)
3	sprigs chopped fresh thyme
½	teaspoon salt
¼	teaspoon black pepper

◉ Heat oven to 350°F. Remove giblets and split hens in half lengthwise. Rinse hens in cold water and pat dry. Place hens in roasting pan skin-side up.

◉ Break the head of garlic into cloves—do not peel—and scatter them around hens. Drizzle hens and garlic with olive oil and lemon juice. Sprinkle hens with thyme, salt, and pepper.

◉ Bake 50 minutes to 1 hour, until juices run clear. The soft garlic can be squeezed from the cloves and spread on crusty bread.

Variation
Herbed Cornish Game Hens: Omit garlic, olive oil, lemon juice, and thyme. Rub hens with 2 teaspoons butter/canola oil blend and sprinkle with 1 teaspoon herbes de Provence, ½ teaspoon rubbed sage, ½ teaspoon salt, and ¼ teaspoon black pepper. Bake as directed above.

Makes 4 servings

Traditional Roast Turkey

1	10- to 12-pound fresh turkey (or if frozen, thawed), giblets and neck removed
1	tablespoon butter/canola oil blend
2	teaspoons rubbed sage
1	teaspoon dried thyme
1	teaspoon dried rosemary
1	teaspoon salt
½	teaspoon black pepper
½	teaspoon paprika

◉ Heat oven to 325°F. Rinse turkey under cold water and pat dry. Place in roasting pan breast side up. Tuck drumsticks under tail skin. Fold wings under back. Rub turkey with butter and sprinkle with seasonings. Cover with an aluminum foil tent. Roast for 2½ hours. Remove foil and roast an additional 1 to 1 ½ hours, until internal temperature reaches 180°F and juices run clear when thigh is pierced with a fork. (Roasting time depends on size of bird—about 20 minutes per pound. Also note that if the bird is stuffed allow an additional 30 minutes roasting time.)

◉ Remove turkey to serving platter and allow to rest 15 minutes before carving. Reserve pan drippings for Pan Gravy (pg. 134), if desired.

Makes 10–12 servings

Sage Stuffing

This recipe will stuff a 10–12 pound turkey. You can also cut the ingredients in half for a large roasting chicken. If you like, you can cube fresh bread the night before and allow it to sit uncovered overnight to get stale.

5	cups stale French bread, cubed
5	cups stale oatmeal or potato bread, cubed
2	tablespoons butter/canola oil blend
1	cup diced onion (about 1 medium onion)
1½	cups diced celery (about 3 ribs)
1	14½-oz. can chicken broth
1½	teaspoons rubbed sage
½	teaspoon dried thyme
½	teaspoon dried rosemary
½	teaspoon salt
¼	teaspoon black pepper

◉ Prepare bread and set aside in a large bowl.

◉ Melt butter in a skillet over medium heat. Add onion and celery and cook about 5–7 minutes, until onion is translucent. Add onion and celery to bread cubes along with remaining ingredients and mix well.

◉ Use to stuff a turkey or chicken or spoon into a 2-quart casserole dish that has been coated with vegetable spray. Cover with aluminum foil and bake in a 350°F oven for 20 minutes. Remove foil and bake an additional 10 minutes.

Makes 10–12 servings

Pan Gravy

Made from pan drippings, this method works well for any roasted poultry or beef.

	Pan drippings
	Canned chicken or beef broth
¼	cup cold water
2	tablespoons all-purpose flour
¼	teaspoon salt
⅛	teaspoon black pepper

◉ Remove roasted poultry or beef from roasting pan. Pour pan drippings into a glass measuring cup and let sit about 3–5 minutes. When the fat has risen to the top, skim of all but about 1 tablespoon. Add chicken or beef broth to measure 2 cups. Add broth and pan drippings back to roasting pan and scrape to loosen the browned bits on the bottom of the pan.

◉ If your roasting pan is top-of-the-stove safe, use it to prepare gravy—if not, use a skillet. Bring broth and drippings to a boil. Shake water and flour together in a lidded jar. Whisk flour slurry into broth mixture in a slow, steady stream. Whisk until thick and bubbly. Season with salt and pepper and cook 1 minute more.

Makes about 2 cups

Plain Omelet

4	large eggs
⅛	teaspoon salt
⅛	teaspoon black pepper

◉ Heat skillet over medium-high heat. Coat with vegetable spray. Beat eggs well with salt and pepper. Pour eggs into skillet. As eggs begin to cook, lift edges slightly with spatula to allow uncooked egg to run underneath. When eggs have set, fold omelet in half, making a crescent shape, or fold in thirds, making a burrito-like shape.

Fillings for omelets: When eggs are almost set, spoon one of the following fillings onto the center of the omelet and fold as above. Cook another 1–2 minutes for eggs to set.

Cheddar and Vegetable Filling: Heat 1 teaspoon canola oil in a skillet over medium-high heat. Add ¼ cup diced onion, ¼ cup diced green bell pepper, and ¼ cup diced celery and cook about 5–7 minutes, until tender. Spoon vegetables onto omelet, sprinkle with ¼ cup shredded sharp Cheddar cheese, and fold.

Southwestern Filling: Spoon ¼ cup canned black beans, rinsed and drained, and ¼ cup Fresh Tomato Salsa (pg. 27) or bottled salsa onto omelet and fold. Serve with a dollop of lite sour cream or plain yogurt.

Tomato and Basil Filling: Sprinkle omelet with 1 medium Roma tomato, diced, and 1 tablespoon thinly sliced fresh basil and fold.

Makes 2 servings

Spinach Frittata

A frittata is essentially a large omelet finished in the oven. It is easy to prepare and is served in wedges straight from the skillet. For lower lactose, choose the Parmesan cheese in this recipe.

1	tablespoon butter/canola oil blend
1	medium onion, sliced thin (about 1 cup)
1	10-oz. package frozen spinach, thawed and squeezed dry
6	large eggs
½	teaspoon salt
¼	teaspoon black pepper
4	ounces crumbled feta cheese or grated Parmesan cheese (about ½ cup)

◉ Heat oven to broil. In an oven-proof skillet, melt butter over medium-high heat. Add onion slices and cook about 5–7 minutes, until tender. Add spinach and cook 1 minute more. Reduce heat to medium.

◉ In a small bowl beat eggs with salt and pepper and pour into skillet. Cover and cook about 7–8 minutes, until almost set. Sprinkle with cheese and place under broiler for 3–5 minutes, until eggs are fully set.

Variations

Mushroom Swiss Frittata: Omit spinach and feta or Parmesan cheese. Add 8 ounces fresh white mushrooms—stems removed and caps sliced—along with the onions. When eggs are almost set, sprinkle with 1 cup Swiss cheese and proceed as directed.

Roasted Red Pepper Frittata: Omit feta cheese. Substitute 1 12-oz. jar roasted red peppers, drained and chopped, for the spinach. Add 2 tablespoons thinly sliced fresh basil with the eggs, salt, and pepper. When eggs are almost set, sprinkle with ½ cup grated Parmesan cheese and proceed as directed.

Makes 4 servings

Black Bean Frittata

1	tablespoon butter/canola oil
½	cup diced onion (about 1 small onion)
1	4-oz. can diced green chiles
1	15-oz. can black beans, rinsed and drained
6	large eggs
¼	teaspoon salt
¼	teaspoon black pepper
¼	teaspoon cumin
½	cup extra-sharp Cheddar cheese
	Fresh Tomato Salsa (pg. 27) or bottled salsa (optional)
	Velvety Guacamole (pg. 28) (optional)
	Lite sour cream or plain yogurt (optional)

◉ Heat oven to broil. In an oven-proof skillet melt butter over medium-high heat. Add onion and cook about 5–7 minutes, until tender. Add chiles and beans and cook 2 minutes more. Reduce heat to medium. Beat eggs with salt, pepper, and cumin and pour into skillet.

◉ Cook about 8–10 minutes, until almost set. Sprinkle with cheese and place under broiler for 3–5 minutes, until eggs are set.

◉ Cut into wedges and serve with Fresh Tomato Salsa (pg. 27) or bottled salsa, Velvety Guacamole (pg. 28), lite sour cream, or plain yogurt, if desired.

Makes 4 servings

Bacon and Cheddar Quiche

If you are lactose intolerant, consider taking a lactase tablet before consuming.

1	recipe 1-crust Standard Pastry Dough (pg. 197)
8	slices center-cut bacon, cooked crisp, drained on paper towels, and crumbled
½	cup diced onion (about 1 small onion)
½	cup diced green bell pepper (about ½ medium pepper)
1	cup shredded sharp Cheddar cheese
5	large eggs
1	cup fat-free half and half
1	cup 2% milk
¼	teaspoon salt
⅛	teaspoon black pepper
⅛	teaspoon paprika

- Heat oven to 425°F. Line a 9-inch pie plate with prepared pastry and crimp edges. Sprinkle with crumbled bacon, onion, bell pepper, and cheese.
- Beat eggs with half and half, milk, salt, and pepper and pour on top of cheese. Sprinkle with paprika. Bake for 15 minutes. Reduce oven temperature to 325°F. Bake an additional 30–35 minutes, until knife inserted near center of quiche comes out clean. Allow to stand 10 minutes before serving.

Variations
Quiche Lorraine: Substitute grated Swiss cheese for the Cheddar.
Crab Quiche: Substitute 8 ounces lump or claw crabmeat, picked over, for the bacon.
Sausage and Mushroom Quiche: Substitute 8 ounces cooked Breakfast Sausage (pg. 117) for the bacon. Substitute 4 ounces fresh white mushrooms, stems removed and caps sliced, for the bell pepper.

Makes 6 servings

Broiled Fish

1½	pounds fresh fish fillets (grouper, haddock, orange roughy, or other firm fish)
1	tablespoon butter/canola oil blend, softened
1	tablespoon fresh lemon juice
½	teaspoon lemon zest (grated rind)
¼	teaspoon salt
⅛	teaspoon black pepper
	Lemon wedges (optional)

◉ Set oven to broil. Coat broiler pan with vegetable spray. Cut fillets, if necessary, into 4 even pieces and place on broiler pan. Mix remaining ingredients together and spread on fillets.

◉ Broil for 10–12 minutes, depending on thickness of fillets, until fish flakes when tested with a fork. Garnish with lemon wedges, if desired.

Makes 4 servings

Oven-Fried Fish Sticks

As a child, I loved those frozen fish sticks with minced who-knows-what inside. With these fish sticks, you know what you're getting. Serve with Tartar Sauce (pg. 189), Cocktail Sauce (pg. 189) or 1000 Island Dressing (pg. 69).

1½	pounds fresh fish fillets (grouper, haddock, mahimahi, or other firm fish)
½	cup all-purpose flour
½	cup plain bread crumbs
2	teaspoons Old Bay seasoning
½	teaspoon garlic powder
½	teaspoon salt
¼	teaspoon black pepper
1	large egg
¼	cup skim or soy milk
	Lemon wedges (optional)

◉ Preheat oven to 450°F. Cut fillets into about 1½-inch strips.

◉ In a shallow bowl combine flour, bread crumbs, Old Bay seasoning, garlic powder, salt, and pepper. In a second shallow bowl whisk together egg and milk.

◉ Coat a baking sheet with vegetable spray. Dip fish strips in egg wash, dredge in flour mixture, and place on prepared baking sheet. Spray fish strips with vegetable spray. Bake for 10–12 minutes, depending on thickness of strips, until fish flakes when tested with a fork. Garnish with lemon wedges, if desired.

Makes 4 servings

Creole Catfish

½   cup all-purpose flour

½   cup cornmeal

1½   tablespoons Creole seasoning*

¼   teaspoon salt

⅛   teaspoon black pepper

1   large egg

¼   cup skim or soy milk

4   6-oz. farm-raised catfish fillets

     Lemon wedges (optional)

◉ Heat oven to 425°F. In a shallow bowl combine flour, cornmeal, Creole seasoning, salt, and pepper. In another shallow bowl whisk together egg and milk.

◉ Coat a baking sheet with vegetable spray. Dip fillets in egg wash, dredge in flour mixture, and place on baking sheet. Spray fillets with vegetable spray. Bake for 12 minutes. Carefully flip fillets with a spatula and bake an additional 10–12 minutes, until fish flakes when tested with a fork. Serve with lemon wedges, if desired.

*If you don't have Creole seasoning on hand, you can make your own using the recipe on page 142.

Makes 4 servings

Creole Seasoning

2	teaspoons garlic powder
1½	teaspoons paprika
1	teaspoon salt
1	teaspoon onion powder
1	teaspoon dried oregano
1	teaspoon dried thyme
1	teaspoon cayenne pepper
1	teaspoon black pepper

◉ Mix ingredients together and store in an airtight container.

Makes about ¼ cup

Rosemary and Lemon Salmon

Salmon is rich in Omega-3 fatty acids, which have anti-inflammatory properties. This quick and easy dish is a delicious way to incorporate these important fatty acids into your diet.

4	salmon fillets (about 1½ pounds)
1	tablespoon olive oil
2	tablespoons fresh lemon juice
1	green onion, chopped fine, or 2 tablespoons fresh chives, snipped
2	tablespoons chopped fresh rosemary or 1 teaspoon dried rosemary
¼	teaspoon salt
⅛	teaspoon black pepper
	Lemon wedges (optional)

◉ Heat oven to 400° F. Coat a 13 x 9 baking dish with vegetable spray. Arrange fillets in dish. Drizzle fish with olive oil and lemon juice. Sprinkle with onion, rosemary, salt, and pepper.

◉ Bake for 15–20 minutes, until fish flakes when tested with a fork. Garnish with lemon wedges, if desired.

Variations

Dill and Lemon Salmon: Substitute 2 tablespoons fresh dill, snipped , or 1 teaspoon dried dill for the rosemary.

Tarragon and Lemon Salmon: Substitute 2 tablespoons fresh tarragon or 1 teaspoon dried tarragon for the rosemary.

Makes 4 servings

Tuna Noodle Casserole

8	ounces egg noodles, cooked to package directions
1	recipe Cheddar Sauce (pg. 164)
2	6-oz. cans albacore tuna, packed in water and drained*
1	7-oz. jar roasted red peppers, drained and chopped
1	cup frozen peas
½	cup plain bread crumbs
1	tablespoon butter/canola oil blend, melted

◉ While the egg noodles cook, prepare Cheddar Sauce.

◉ Preheat oven to 350°F. Combine noodles, Cheddar Sauce, tuna, roasted red peppers, and peas in a large bowl and mix well. Spoon into a 2-quart casserole dish. Combine bread crumbs and butter and sprinkle on top of casserole. Bake 25–30 minutes until bubbly.

*If concerned about mercury levels in albacore tuna because of pregnancy or if preparing for children, substitute chunk light tuna.

Makes 6 servings

Garlic Shrimp Linguine

8	ounces linguine, cooked to package directions
1	tablespoon butter
1	tablespoon olive oil
2	teaspoons minced garlic (about 4 medium cloves)
1	tablespoon fresh lemon juice
¼	cup chardonnay
½	teaspoon Old Bay seasoning
¼	teaspoon salt
1	pound large shrimp, peeled, deveined, and tails removed
	Lemon wedges (optional)

◉ While pasta cooks, heat butter and olive oil in a large skillet over medium heat. Add garlic and cook 1 minute. Add lemon juice, wine, Old Bay seasoning, salt, and shrimp.

◉ Cook 3–5 minutes, until shrimp turn pink. Spoon shrimp with sauce over hot linguine. Garnish with lemon wedges, if desired.

Makes 4 servings

Crab Cakes

Serve these classic crab cakes with lemon wedges and a dollop of Tartar Sauce (pg. 189) or 1000 Island Dressing (pg. 69).

1	pound lump crabmeat, picked over
1	cup plain bread crumbs
1	large egg, slightly beaten
¼	cup finely diced onion (about ½ small onion)
¼	cup finely diced red bell pepper (about ¼ medium pepper)
1	tablespoon Miracle Whip
1	tablespoon fresh lemon juice
1	teaspoon Old Bay seasoning
½	teaspoon salt
¼	teaspoon black pepper
¼	teaspoon dry mustard

- Heat oven to 400°F. Place all ingredients into a large bowl and gently fold together to combine.

- Coat baking sheet with vegetable spray. Shape crab cake mixture into 8 patties and place on prepared sheet. Bake for 10 minutes. Gently flip patties over with a spatula and bake an additional 5–7 minutes, until golden brown.

Makes 4 main-dish servings or 8 appetizers

Scallop and Feta Bake

1	tablespoon olive oil
1	medium green bell pepper, cut into thin strips
1	medium onion, sliced thin
1	teaspoon minced garlic (about 2 medium cloves)
1	14½-oz. can diced tomatoes
1	pound medium-sized sea scallops
8–10	kalamata olives, pitted and halved
½	teaspoon salt
¼	teaspoon black pepper
4	ounces feta cheese, crumbled
8	ounces linguine, cooked to package directions

◉ Heat oven to 425°F. Heat oil in a skillet over medium-high heat. Add bell pepper and onion and cook about 5 minutes. Add garlic and cook 1 minute more. Add tomatoes and heat through.

◉ Coat a 2-quart casserole dish with vegetable spray. Spoon half of the tomato sauce into casserole. Arrange scallops on top of sauce. Spoon remaining sauce on top of scallops.

◉ Sprinkle with olives, salt, pepper, and feta cheese. Bake for 18–20 minutes, until scallops are opaque. Serve over hot linguine.

Makes 4 servings

Skillet-Fried Shrimp

Know anyone who doesn't like fried shrimp? Serve these lightly fried beauties with lemon wedges, Tartar Sauce (pg. 189), and/or Cocktail Sauce (pg. 189). Another favorite of mine is double dipping in Texas Pete's Wing Sauce and Blue Cheese Dressing (pg. 66).

1	cup all-purpose flour
2	teaspoons Old Bay seasoning
1	teaspoon garlic powder
½	teaspoon salt
¼	teaspoon black pepper
1	large egg
¼	cup skim or soy milk
3	tablespoons canola oil, divided
1	pound large shrimp, peeled, deveined, and tail left intact

- In a shallow bowl combine flour, Old Bay seasoning, garlic powder, salt, and pepper and mix well. In another shallow bowl whisk together egg and milk.

- Heat 1½ tablespoons oil in skillet over medium-high heat. Working in 2 batches, dip shrimp in egg wash, dredge in flour mixture, and place in skillet. Cook about 2–3 minutes, turn shrimp over and cook an additional 2–3 minutes, until shrimp have curled up and are golden. Remove shrimp and drain on paper towels. Add remaining 1½ tablespoons oil to skillet and repeat with remaining shrimp.

Makes 4 servings

Shrimp Creole

2	tablespoons olive or canola oil
1	cup diced onion (about 1 medium onion)
1	cup diced green bell pepper (about 1 medium pepper)
1	cup sliced celery (about 2 ribs)
1	teaspoon minced garlic (about 2 medium cloves)
1	14½-oz. can crushed tomatoes
6	tablespoons tomato paste
2	bay leaves
2	teaspoons Creole seasoning*
1½	pounds large shrimp, peeled, deveined, and tails removed
	Hot jasmine or white rice

◉ Heat oil in a Dutch oven over medium-high heat. Add onions, bell pepper, and celery and cook about 5 minutes. Add garlic and cook 1 minute. Add tomatoes, tomato paste, bay leaves, and Creole seasoning and bring to a boil. Reduce heat, cover, and simmer about 30–35 minutes.

◉ Add shrimp and simmer about 5–7 minutes, until shrimp turn pink. Discard bay leaves before serving. Serve over hot jasmine or white rice.

*If you don't have Creole seasoning on hand, you can make your own using the recipe on page 142.

Makes 6 servings

Steamed Clams

2	dozen Littleneck clams, scrubbed
½	cup chardonnay
1	tablespoon fresh lemon juice
1	teaspoon minced garlic (about 2 medium cloves)
	Lemon wedges
	Crusty bread

◉ Place the clams, chardonnay, lemon juice, and garlic in a large skillet and bring to a boil. Reduce heat, cover, and simmer 5–10 minutes, until shells open. Discard any clams that have not opened. Serve with lemon wedges and crusty bread for dipping in broth.

Makes 2 servings

Beef Lasagna

If you are lactose intolerant, substitute silken soft tofu for the ricotta and silken firm tofu or sharp Cheddar cheese for the mozzarella.

1	15-oz. container part-skim ricotta cheese
2	cups shredded part-skim mozzarella cheese
¼	cup grated Parmesan cheese, plus 2 tablespoons
1	large egg
1½	teaspoons Italian seasoning
¼	teaspoon black pepper
5	cups Tomato Beef Sauce (pg. 162)
12	lasagna noodles, cooked to package directions

◉ Preheat oven to 350°F. Combine ricotta, mozzarella, ¼ cup Parmesan, egg, Italian seasoning and pepper in a bowl and mix well.

◉ Spread 2 cups of sauce in the bottom of a 13 x 9 baking dish. Arrange 4 lasagna noodles on top of sauce. Spoon ½ of the cheese mixture on top of noodles. Spoon 1 cup of sauce on top of cheese. Repeat layers of noodles, cheese, sauce and noodles again. Top with remaining sauce. Sprinkle with remaining 2 tablespoons Parmesan.

◉ Cover with foil and bake 30 minutes. Uncover and bake an additional 15 minutes.

◉ Allow to cool 15 minutes before serving.

Makes 10 servings

Spaghetti with Meatballs

1¼	pounds lean hamburger
¼	cup finely diced onion
¼	cup finely diced green bell pepper
½	cup plain bread crumbs
1	large egg
2	teaspoons Worcestershire sauce
1	teaspoon Italian seasoning
½	teaspoon minced garlic (about 1 medium clove)
¼	teaspoon salt
⅛	teaspoon black pepper
4	cups Marinara Sauce (pg. 163) or bottled sauce
12	ounces spaghetti, cooked to package directions
	Grated Parmesan cheese

- Preheat oven to 375°F. In a large bowl combine hamburger, onion, bell pepper, bread crumbs, egg, Worcestershire sauce, Italian seasoning, garlic, salt, and pepper and mix well.

- Roll beef mixture into 2-inch balls and place on a baking sheet. Bake for 25–30 minutes, until no longer pink inside.

- While meatballs are in the oven, prepare sauce. Add meatballs to sauce and simmer 15–20 minutes. While meatballs are simmering, prepare spaghetti.

- Serve meatballs and sauce over pasta. Garnish with grated Parmesan cheese, if desired.

Makes 6 servings

Stuffed Shells Florentine

For a lower lactose recipe, substitute silken soft tofu for the ricotta and silken firm tofu or sharp Cheddar cheese for the mozzarella.

1	12-oz. package jumbo shell pasta, cooked to package directions
1	10-oz. package frozen chopped spinach, thawed and squeezed dry
1	15-oz. container part-skim ricotta cheese
1	cup shredded part-skim mozzarella cheese
¼	cup grated Parmesan cheese
1	large egg
2	teaspoons Italian seasoning
¼	teaspoon black pepper
3	cups Marinara Sauce (pg. 163), Tomato Beef Sauce (pg. 162), or bottled sauce
¼	cup grated Parmesan cheese

◉ Preheat oven to 350°F. While pasta is cooling, combine spinach, ricotta, mozzarella, ¼ cup Parmesan, egg, Italian seasoning, and pepper in a bowl and mix well.

◉ Spoon half of the sauce into a 13 x 9-inch baking dish. Stuff shells with cheese mixture (about 2 tablespoons each) and arrange in a single layer, open side down, on top of sauce. Spoon remaining sauce on top of shells. Sprinkle with remaining ¼ cup Parmesan cheese.

◉ Cover with foil and bake 30 minutes. Remove foil and bake an additional 10 minutes.

◉ Let stand 10–15 minutes before serving.

Makes 8 servings

Fettuccini Alfredo

Fettuccini Alfredo can be prepared in minutes and can be served as a side dish or as an entrée when topped with cooked chicken breast, shrimp, or scallops. I have tried several soy products as substitutions for the dairy in this dish without much luck. So if you are lactose intolerant, I suggest a lactase tablet beforehand.

1	pound fettuccini, cooked to package directions
2	tablespoons butter/canola oil blend
2	tablespoons all-purpose flour
1½	cups fat-free half and half
¾–1	cup skim milk
¼	teaspoon black pepper
¾	cup grated Parmesan cheese

◉ While pasta cooks, melt butter in a large skillet over medium-high heat. Whisk in flour and cook 1 minute, whisking constantly, until smooth. Whisk in half and half in a slow, steady stream. Whisk in ¾ cup milk. Bring to a boil. Reduce heat and simmer 3–5 minutes, whisking occasionally, until sauce has thickened.

◉ Add pepper and Parmesan and whisk until smooth. If sauce is thicker than desired, thin with ¼ cup milk. Serve sauce over hot pasta.

Makes 6–8 servings

Fettuccini Alfredo with Garden Vegetables

1	recipe Fettuccini Alfredo (pg. 154)
2	tablespoons olive oil
1	medium onion, sliced thin
½	medium green bell pepper, sliced in thin strips
½	medium red bell pepper, sliced in thin strips
1	small zucchini, ends removed and sliced thin
4	ounces cremini mushrooms, stems removed and caps sliced
1	teaspoon minced garlic (about 2 medium cloves)
¼	teaspoon salt
⅛	teaspoon black pepper
10–12	kalamata olives, pitted and halved

◉ Prepare Fettuccini Alfredo.

◉ Heat olive oil in a large skillet over medium-high heat. Add onion and green and red bell pepper and cook about 3 minutes. Add zucchini and mushrooms and cook another 4–5 minutes, until vegetables are tender. Add garlic, salt, pepper, and olives and cook 1 minute more.

◉ Serve atop pasta and sauce.

Makes 6–8 servings

Fettuccini with Fresh Basil and Feta

8	ounces fettuccini, cooked to package directions
4	ounces feta cheese, crumbled
¼	cup fresh basil leaves, sliced or torn
1	tablespoon olive oil
1	teaspoon minced garlic (about 2 medium cloves)
3	medium Roma tomatoes, diced
16	kalamata olives, pitted and halved
¼	teaspoon salt
⅛	teaspoon black pepper

◉ Drain fettuccini and place in a large serving bowl with crumbled feta and basil.

◉ Heat olive oil in a skillet over medium-high heat. Add garlic and cook 1 minute. Add tomatoes, olives, salt, and pepper and cook about 2–3 minutes to heat through.

◉ Add tomato mixture to fettuccini and toss well to coat.

Makes 4 servings

Carbonara

Pancetta is an Italian bacon that is not smoked and is available in the deli section of many grocery stores. If you are lactose intolerant, omit the half and half—it will be just as tasty.

1	pound fettuccini or linguini, cooked to package directions
8	slices pancetta or center-cut bacon, chopped
1	teaspoon minced garlic (about 2 medium cloves)
½	cup fat-free half and half
¾	cup grated Parmesan cheese, plus more for garnish
2	tablespoons flat leaf parsley, chopped
¼	teaspoon black pepper

◉ While pasta cooks, place pancetta or bacon in skillet over medium heat and cook until crisp, about 5 minutes. Add garlic and cook 1 minute more.

◉ In a large serving bowl combine drained pasta, pancetta, half and half, ¾ cup Parmesan, parsley, and pepper and toss well to coat.

◉ Garnish with extra grated Parmesan, if desired.

Makes 6 servings

Pasta Primavera

8	ounces bowtie, rotini, shell, or other shaped pasta, cooked to package directions
2	tablespoons olive oil
½	medium red bell pepper, cut into thin strips
½	medium yellow bell pepper, cut into thin strips
½	green bell pepper, cut into thin strips
1	medium onion, sliced thin
4	ounces fresh white or cemini mushrooms, stems removed and caps sliced
1	small zucchini or yellow squash, ends removed, halved lengthwise and sliced
½	cup sun-dried tomatoes (packed in oil or reconstituted), sliced
1	cup frozen peas, thawed
1½	teaspoons minced garlic, about 3 medium cloves
½	cup grated Parmesan cheese, plus more for garnish
¼	cup fresh basil leaves, sliced or torn
1	teaspoon Italian seasoning
¼	teaspoon salt
⅛	teaspoon black pepper

- While pasta cooks, heat olive oil in a large skillet over medium-high heat. Add red, yellow, and green bell pepper and onion and cook about 5 minutes. Add mushrooms and zucchini and cook another 3 minutes. Add sun-dried tomatoes, peas, and garlic and cook an additional 2–3 minutes.

- In a large serving bowl combine drained pasta, vegetables, Parmesan, basil, Italian seasoning, salt, and pepper and toss well to coat. Garnish with additional grated Parmesan, if desired.

Makes 4 servings

Chicken Linguini
with Tomato Cream Sauce

8	ounces linguini, cooked to package directions
½	cup chicken broth
½	cup sun-dried tomatoes (not oil-packed)
1	tablespoon olive oil
1	cup diced onion (about 1 medium onion)
½	teaspoon minced garlic (about 1 medium clove)
1	pound boneless, skinless chicken breast, cut into 1- to 1½-inch strips
½	teaspoon Italian seasoning
¼	teaspoon salt
⅛	teaspoon black pepper
½	cup fat-free half and half or soy milk
1	tablespoon fresh basil leaves, sliced thin

◉ While the pasta cooks, heat chicken broth to boiling in a small saucepan. Remove from heat, add sun-dried tomatoes, and set aside.

◉ Heat olive oil in a skillet over medium-high heat. Add onion and cook about 5 minutes. Add garlic and cook 1 minute more. Add chicken strips, Italian seasoning, salt, and pepper and cook until chicken is browned, about 5 minutes.

◉ Chop the sun-dried tomatoes and add to skillet along with the broth and bring to a boil. Reduce heat, cover, and simmer about 10 minutes, until chicken is no longer pink inside.

◉ Stir in half and half and simmer 3–5 minutes, until sauce has slightly thickened.

◉ Serve over hot linguini and garnish with sliced basil.

Makes 4 servings

Linguini with Clam Sauce

8	ounces linguini, cooked to package directions
1	tablespoon olive oil
½	cup diced onion (about 1 small onion)
1	teaspoon minced garlic (about 2 medium cloves)
2	medium Roma tomatoes, diced
2	10-oz. cans whole baby clams, drained and liquid reserved
½	cup chardonnay
½	teaspoon Italian seasoning
¼	teaspoon salt
⅛	teaspoon black pepper
⅛	teaspoon Old Bay seasoning

◉ While the pasta cooks, heat oil in a skillet over medium heat. Add onion and cook about 5 minutes. Add garlic and cook 1 minute more. Add tomatoes, reserved clam liquid, wine, Italian seasoning, salt, pepper, and Old Bay seasoning and bring to a boil. Reduce heat, cover, and simmer 10 minutes. Add clams and cook 2 minutes more to heat through.

◉ Place cooked pasta in a large serving bowl. Pour clam sauce over pasta and toss well to coat.

Makes 4 servings

Mac and Cheese

The ultimate comfort food for children and adults alike. Consider taking a lactase tablet with this dish as it is not low lactose.

8	ounces elbow macaroni, cooked to package directions
2	tablespoons butter/canola oil blend
½	cup diced onion (about 1 small onion)
1	teaspoon minced garlic (about 2 medium cloves)
2	tablespoons all-purpose flour
1	cup fat-free half and half
1	cup skim milk
½	teaspoon salt
¼	teaspoon black pepper
1½	cups shredded extra-sharp Cheddar cheese
¼	cup grated Parmesan cheese
¼	teaspoon paprika

◉ Preheat oven to 350°F. While the pasta cooks, melt butter in a large skillet over medium-high heat. Add onion and cook about 5 minutes. Add garlic and cook 1 minute more. Whisk in flour and cook about 1 minute, until the mixture has a smooth consistency. Whisk in half and half in a slow and steady stream. Whisk in milk, bring to a boil, and boil 1 minute. Reduce heat and simmer 3–5 minutes, until sauce thickens. Add salt, pepper, and Cheddar and whisk until cheese has melted and sauce is smooth and creamy. Add drained pasta and mix well to coat.

◉ Spoon mac and cheese into a 2-quart casserole dish coated with vegetable spray. Top with Parmesan and paprika. Bake for 30–35 minutes, until golden and bubbly. Let stand 10–15 minutes before serving.

Makes 4–6 servings

Tomato Beef Sauce

This sauce freezes well or can be stored in the refrigerator for up to 5 days.

1½	pounds lean hamburger
2	cups diced onion (about 1 large onion)
½	cup diced green bell pepper (about ½ medium pepper)
½	cup diced red bell pepper (about ½ medium pepper)
1	teaspoon minced garlic (about 2 medium cloves)
4	ounces fresh white mushrooms, stem removed and caps sliced
2	14½-oz. cans diced tomatoes
1	6-oz. can tomato paste
1	8-oz. can tomato sauce
2	bay leaves
2	teaspoons Italian seasoning
1	teaspoon sugar
1	teaspoon salt
½	teaspoon black pepper
½	teaspoon dried oregano

◉ In a Dutch oven cook hamburger, onion, and green and red bell peppers over medium-high heat until beef is browned and vegetables are tender, about 7–8 minutes.

◉ Add garlic and mushrooms and cook another 2 minutes. Add remaining ingredients, stirring well to combine, and bring to a boil. Reduce heat, cover, and simmer about 1 hour, stirring occasionally. Remove bay leaves.

◉ Serve over hot pasta or use in your favorite recipe.

Makes 7–8 cups

Marinara Sauce

This sauce comes together in minutes and is delicious over hot pasta with a sprinkling of grated Parmesan or Romano cheese.

1	tablespoon olive oil
1	cup diced onion (about 1 medium onion)
½	cup diced green bell pepper (about ½ medium pepper)
1	teaspoon minced garlic (about 2 medium cloves)
2	14½-oz. cans diced tomatoes
3	tablespoons tomato paste
½	teaspoon Italian seasoning
½	teaspoon sugar
½	teaspoon salt
¼	teaspoon black pepper
2	tablespoons fresh basil leaves, torn or sliced (optional)

◉ Heat olive oil in a large skillet or Dutch oven over medium heat. Add onion and bell pepper and cook about 5 minutes. Add garlic and cook 1 minute more. Add tomatoes, tomato paste, Italian seasoning, sugar, salt, and pepper and bring to a boil. Reduce heat, cover, and simmer, stirring occasionally, about 25 minutes. Stir in basil, if using, and cook 1 minute more.

◉ Serve over hot pasta.

Makes 3½–4 cups

White Sauce (Bechamel)

This simple sauce is easy to prepare and is the base for many other sauces.

2	tablespoons butter/canola oil blend
2	tablespoons all-purpose flour
1	cup 2% or skim milk
¼	teaspoon salt
⅛	teaspoon black pepper

◉ Melt butter in a skillet or heavy saucepan over medium heat. Whisk in flour and cook 1 minute, whisking constantly. Whisk in milk in a slow and steady stream. Bring to a simmer and cook 3–5 minutes, whisking occasionally, until thickened. Remove from heat and season with salt and pepper.

Variations

Dijon Mustard Sauce: While simmering, whisk in 1 tablespoon Dijon mustard.
Cheddar Sauce: Before removing from heat, whisk in 1 cup shredded sharp Cheddar cheese until melted.
Mornay Sauce: Before removing from heat, whisk in ⅓ cup shredded Swiss cheese and ⅓ cup grated Parmesan cheese until melted.
Velouté Sauce: Substitute chicken broth for the milk.

Makes 1 cup

Pesto

2   cups fresh basil, flat-leafed parsley, or baby spinach

½   cup grated Parmesan or Romano cheese

1   tablespoon minced garlic (about 6 medium cloves)

½   teaspoon salt

¼   cup olive oil

◉ Combine all ingredients except the olive oil in a blender or food processor and blend (or pulse) until smooth, about 1–2 minutes. With machine running, add olive oil slowly and blend until mixture is a smooth consistency.

◉ Serve on warm, crusty bread or toss ⅓ cup with 8 ounces hot pasta to make 4 side dishes.

Makes 1 cup

Italian Seasoning

1   tablespoon dried basil

1   tablespoon dried oregano

1   tablespoon dried rosemary

1   tablespoon dried thyme

1½   teaspoons rubbed sage

1½   teaspoons marjoram

◉ Mix ingredients together and store in an airtight container.

Makes about ⅓ cup

Tips on Dining Out

◉ Don't be afraid to ask your server questions about how dishes are prepared. It is part of his/her job to know or to find out from the chef for you. **Examples**: Is the fish broiled or sauteed in butter? Is the potato salad made fresh on the premises or is it prepackaged? Is it made with mayonnaise or salad dressing?

◉ Don't be afraid to make special requests. Servers understand that people have different dietary needs whether because of illness or dieting. **Examples**: Order salad dressing, butter, sour cream, and other condiments on the side so you can control the fat content. Substitute a baked potato for french fries on a sandwich platter or order items á la carte.

◉ Control portion. Many restaurants serve larger portions then are necessary. **Suggestions**: Eat half and take the rest home for a second meal, or simply leave the food on your plate without feeling guilty. Order an appetizer with salad or soup as your meal rather than an entree.

◉ I don't advise eating at fast-food restaurants on a regular basis because the food is generally high in fat. Sometimes it's unavoidable—shopping with friends, having lunch with co-workers or traveling—and an occasional meal can be okay if you make informed choices. Most of the larger chains offer a nutritional breakdown of items on their menu either on a poster within the restaurant or in pamphlet form. You can also find this information before you go by visiting their Web sites.

◉ Be prepared. Bring along the medicine your doctor has recommended for acid control and/or reducing gas such as Pepcid AC or Beano.

Red Potatoes with Rosemary

2	pounds small red potatoes
½	teaspoon salt
1	tablespoon butter/canola oil blend
1	tablespoon chopped fresh rosemary
½	teaspoon salt
¼	teaspoon black pepper

◉ Wash potatoes and cut in half if necessary to make them approximately the same size and place in large saucepan. Add enough water to cover potatoes and ½ teaspoon salt.

◉ Bring to a boil. Boil about 20 minutes, until fork-tender. Drain and return potatoes to saucepan. Add butter, rosemary, salt, and pepper and toss to coat.

Makes 6 servings

Basic Mashed Potatoes

2	pounds all-purpose or Yukon Gold potatoes
$\frac{1}{2}$	teaspoon salt
2	tablespoons butter/canola oil blend
$\frac{1}{2}$–$\frac{3}{4}$ cup	2% milk or chicken broth
$\frac{1}{2}$	teaspoon salt
$\frac{1}{4}$	teaspoon black pepper

◉ Peel potatoes, cut in half, and place in a large saucepan. Add enough water to cover potatoes. Add ½ teaspoon salt and bring to a boil. Boil 20–25 minutes, until potatoes are fork-tender. Drain and return potatoes to saucepan.

◉ Mash potatoes slightly with hand mixer or potato masher. Add butter and ½ cup milk and mash until desired consistency, 1–2 minutes, adding more milk if necessary. Season with salt and pepper and mash 10–15 seconds to blend.

Variations
Garlic Mashed Potatoes: Add 6–8 peeled medium cloves of garlic to the potatoes before boiling.
Horseradish Mashed Potatoes: Add 1 tablespoon prepared horseradish along with the butter and milk.
Herbed Mashed Potatoes: Blend in 1 tablespoon fresh basil, rosemary, or thyme with the salt and pepper.

Makes 6 servings

Oven Fries

Fries baked in the oven are so much healthier than their deep-fried counterparts because of the small amount of oil used. You can vary the seasoning if you wish by substituting garlic powder, onion powder, chili powder, or any number of dried herbs for the Italian seasoning.

3	large baking potatoes
1½	tablespoons canola or olive oil
1	teaspoon Italian seasoning
½	teaspoon salt
⅛	teaspoon black pepper
⅛	teaspoon paprika

◉ Preheat oven to 450°F. Wash potatoes and cut in half lengthwise. Cut each half of potato lengthwise into 4 wedges. Place potato wedges and oil in a large ziplock bag; seal and shake to coat.

◉ Coat a baking sheet with vegetable spray. Arrange potato wedges on baking sheet in a single layer. Sprinkle with seasonings. Bake for 15 minutes. Turn potatoes with a spatula. Bake about 15–20 minutes more, until potatoes are crispy outside and tender inside.

Makes 4–6 servings

Scalloped Potatoes

This recipe is the first step-by-step cooking lesson I had with my mom, and I remember it like it was yesterday. I've altered her version only slightly so that it contains less saturated fat.

3	tablespoons all-purpose flour
1	teaspoon salt
½	teaspoon black pepper
2	pounds all-purpose potatoes (about 6 medium potatoes), peeled and sliced thin
2	medium onions, halved and sliced thin, divided
3	tablespoons butter/canola oil blend, divided
1½–2 cups 2% or soy milk	
¼	teaspoon paprika

◉ Preheat oven to 350°F. Coat a 2-quart casserole dish with vegetable spray.

◉ Combine flour, salt, and pepper in a small bowl and mix well. Arrange one-third of the potato slices in prepared pan. Top with half of the onion slices. Dot with 1 tablespoon butter broken into 3 or 4 pieces. Sprinkle with half of the flour mixture.

◉ Repeat layers of one-third of the potato slices, remaining onion slices, 1 tablespoon butter, and remaining flour. Top with remaining potato slices and dot with remaining 1 tablespoon butter.

◉ Pour milk over top until just covering potatoes. Sprinkle with paprika.

◉ Cover with foil and bake 1 hour. Remove foil and bake about 30 minutes more, until potatoes are fork-tender. Let stand 10–15 minutes before serving.

Variation
Au Gratin Potatoes: Sprinkle the first two layers of potatoes with ½ cup shredded sharp Cheddar cheese (regular or 2%) each.

Makes 6 servings

Mashed Sweet Potatoes

2   pounds sweet potatoes (about 6 medium sweet potatoes), peeled and quartered

1   tablespoon butter/canola oil blend

¼   cup brown sugar

½   teaspoon salt

¼   teaspoon ground ginger

¼   teaspoon ground nutmeg

◉ Place potatoes in a large saucepan and add enough water to cover. Bring to a boil and boil about 25–30 minutes, until fork-tender. Drain and return potatoes to saucepan.

◉ Mash potatoes slightly with hand mixer or potato masher. Add butter, brown sugar, salt, ginger, and nutmeg and mash to desired consistency, 1–2 minutes.

Makes 4–6 servings

Roasted Root Vegetables

8	medium carrots, cut into 2-inch pieces
10–12	red potatoes, washed and cut in half
3	medium onions, quartered
1	rib celery, sliced (about ½ cup)
2	tablespoons olive oil
2	teaspoons herbes de Provence
1	teaspoon salt
¼	teaspoon black pepper

◉ Preheat oven to 375°F. Place carrots, potatoes, onions, and celery in a 9 x 13-inch baking dish or roasting pan. Drizzle with olive oil and toss to coat. Sprinkle with seasonings.

◉ Bake about 1 hour, stirring after 30 minutes, until vegetables are tender.

Makes 6 servings

Winter Squash Bake

2	medium acorn or butternut squash, halved lengthwise and seeded
4	teaspoons butter/canola oil blend
4	teaspoons dark brown sugar
$\frac{1}{2}$	teaspoon salt
$\frac{1}{8}$	teaspoon black pepper

◉ Preheat oven to 350°F. Arrange squash in baking dish cut side up. Dot each half with 1 teaspoon butter and 1 teaspoon brown sugar. Sprinkle with salt and pepper. Add about ½ inch of water to the baking dish. Bake about 1 hour, until fork-tender.

Variation

Apple Spice Squash: Omit pepper. After arranging squash in baking dish, peel, core, and chop 1 large baking apple (e.g., Cortland, Jonathan, or Rome Beauty) and spoon evenly into squash halves. Dot with butter and brown sugar. Sprinkle with salt, ¼ teaspoon cinnamon, and ⅛ teaspoon ground nutmeg.

Makes 4 servings

Maple-Glazed Carrots

1	pound baby-cut carrots
2	tablespoons pure maple syrup
1	tablespoon butter/canola oil blend
½	teaspoon orange zest (grated rind)
¼	teaspoon ground nutmeg

◉ Place carrots in a medium saucepan with 1 inch of water. Bring to a boil and boil about 15 minutes, until fork-tender. Drain and return carrots to pan.

◉ Stir in maple syrup, butter, orange zest, and nutmeg and cook 1–2 minutes over medium heat, until butter has melted and carrots are well coated.

Variation
Glazed Carrots with Ginger: Substitute brown sugar for the maple syrup. Substitute 1 teaspoon peeled and grated fresh gingerroot for the orange zest. Substitute salt for the nutmeg.

Makes 4 servings

Carrots and Peas with Fresh Thyme

1	pound baby-cut carrots
1	10-oz. package frozen peas, thawed
1	tablespoon butter/canola oil blend
1	tablespoon chopped fresh thyme
¼	teaspoon salt
⅛	teaspoon black pepper

◉ Place carrots in a large saucepan with 1 inch of water. Bring to a boil and boil about 15 minutes, until fork-tender.

◉ Add peas and cook 2–3 minutes to heat through. Drain and return to pan. Add butter, fresh thyme, salt, and pepper and toss to coat.

Makes 6–8 servings

Peas and Pasta

8	ounces fettuccini or linguine, cooked to package directions
2	teaspoons olive oil
½	teaspoon minced garlic (about 1 medium clove)
½	cup chicken broth
2	tablespoons chopped sun-dried tomatoes (packed in oil or reconstituted)
2	cups frozen peas, thawed
¼	teaspoon salt
⅛	teaspoon black pepper
⅓	cup grated Parmesan cheese

◉ Prepare pasta and drain.

◉ Heat olive oil in a large skillet over medium heat. Add garlic and cook 1 minute. Add broth and sun-dried tomatoes and bring to a boil. Add peas, salt, and pepper and cook about 3 minutes. Add pasta to skillet and toss.

◉ Remove to a serving platter and top with grated Parmesan.

Makes 4 servings

Fresh Green Beans with Feta and Basil

To lower the lactose in this dish, substitute soft tofu for the feta.

1½	pounds fresh green beans, ends trimmed
¼	cup chopped sun-dried tomatoes (packed in oil or reconstituted)
2	teaspoons olive oil
4	ounces feta cheese, crumbled
¼	cup torn or sliced fresh basil
½	teaspoon dried oregano
½	teaspoon salt
¼	teaspoon black pepper

◉ Place green beans in a Dutch oven with 1 inch of water and bring to a boil. Cover and boil about 8–10 minutes, until tender. Drain.

◉ In a serving bowl combine beans with remaining ingredients and toss gently.

Makes 6 servings

Spinach Artichoke Casserole with Roasted Red Peppers

If lactose intolerant, opt for the Miracle Whip instead of the cream cheese.

2	10-oz. packages frozen chopped spinach, thawed and squeezed dry
1	13¾-oz. can artichoke hearts, drained and chopped
1	7-oz. jar roasted red peppers, drained and chopped
½	cup diced onion (about 1 small)
½	cup grated Parmesan cheese
4	ounces reduced-fat cream cheese, softened, or ½ cup Miracle Whip
½	cup 2% or soy milk
¼	teaspoon salt
¼	teaspoon black pepper

◉ Preheat oven to 350°F. Coat a 2-quart casserole dish with vegetable spray.

◉ Combine all ingredients in a large bowl and mix well. Spoon into prepared dish and bake 25–30 minutes, until bubbly. Allow to stand 5 minutes before serving.

Makes 8 servings

Broiled Romas

¼	cup plain bread crumbs
¼	cup grated Parmesan cheese
½	teaspoon minced garlic (about 1 medium clove)
¼	teaspoon Italian seasoning
⅛	teaspoon black pepper
6	Roma tomatoes, halved lengthwise and seeds removed
1	tablespoon olive oil

◉ Set oven to broil. In a small bowl combine bread crumbs, Parmesan cheese, garlic, Italian seasoning, and pepper and mix well.

◉ Coat broiler pan with vegetable spray and arrange tomatoes cut side up on pan. Spoon about 2 teaspoons of the bread crumb mixture onto each Roma half. Drizzle with olive oil. Broil 3–5 minutes, until golden.

Makes 4–6 servings

Triple-Pepper Sauté

This colorful side dish complements any type of meat and is full of antioxidants, the chemicals found naturally in plants that lower the risk of some cancers.

2	tablespoons olive oil
1	medium red bell pepper, cut into thin strips
1	medium green bell pepper, cut into thin strips
1	medium yellow bell pepper, cut into thin strips
1	large onion, halved and sliced thin
1	teaspoon minced garlic (about 2 medium cloves)
½	teaspoon salt
¼	teaspoon black pepper
1	tablespoon chopped or torn fresh basil (optional)

◉ Heat oil in a large skillet over medium-high heat. Add the red, green, and yellow bell pepper and cook about 5 minutes, stirring frequently. Add onion slices and cook, stirring frequently, another 5–7 minutes, until vegetables are tender.

◉ Add garlic, salt, and pepper and cook 1 minute more. Remove to serving dish and top with basil, if desired.

Variation
Triple-Pepper Sauté with Zucchini and Sun-dried Tomatoes: Add 1 small zucchini, ends trimmed and sliced thin, and ¼ cup chopped sun-dried tomatoes (packed in oil or reconstituted) along with the sliced onions.

Makes 4 servings

Skillet-Fried Zucchini

1	large egg
½	cup all-purpose flour
½	cup dry bread crumbs
2	tablespoons grated Parmesan cheese
½	teaspoon Italian seasoning
⅛	teaspoon black pepper
2	tablespoons olive oil, divided
4	small zucchini, ends trimmed and cut in ½-inch slices

◉ Crack egg into bowl and beat slightly.

◉ In a shallow bowl combine flour, bread crumbs, Parmesan cheese, Italian seasoning, and black pepper and mix well.

◉ Heat 1 tablespoon olive oil in skillet over medium-high heat. Dip zucchini slices in egg, dredge in flour mixture, and place in skillet. Cook about 2 minutes on each side, until golden. Remove from skillet and drain on paper towels.

◉ Add remaining oil and repeat with remaining zucchini slices.

Makes 4 servings

Stuffed Zucchini

4	medium zucchini
1	tablespoon olive oil
½	teaspoon salt
¼	teaspoon black pepper
2	Roma tomatoes, diced
¼	cup diced onion (about ½ small)
¼	cup grated Parmesan cheese
¾	cup plain bread crumbs
1	teaspoon minced garlic (about 2 medium cloves)
½	teaspoon Italian seasoning
1	tablespoon olive oil

◉ Preheat oven to 350°F. Trim ends of zucchini and cut lengthwise. Scoop out some of the center of each zucchini half to make a reservoir for the stuffing.

◉ Coat a baking sheet with vegetable spray and arrange zucchini halves on it cut side up. Drizzle with 1 tablespoon olive oil and sprinkle with salt and pepper.

◉ Combine tomatoes, onion, Parmesan cheese, bread crumbs, garlic, and Italian seasoning in a bowl and mix well. Spoon tomato mixture onto zucchini halves evenly. Drizzle with 1 tablespoon olive oil. Bake 25–30 minutes, until golden.

Makes 4 servings

What to Look for on Food Labels

- Check serving size and number of servings per container—it can be misleading. For example, 1 packaged muffin or "single-serve" bag of potato chips may actually be considered 2 or more servings.

- Check amounts of total fat and the breakdown of those fats: saturated, monounsaturated, polyunsaturated, and trans fats.

- Check sodium amounts, especially when looking at foods labeled low-fat. Often the product contains more sodium (to enhance the flavor) to make up for the reduction of fat.

- Check dietary fiber. Labels are not required to break down fiber into soluble and insoluble, but you will have a better idea of how much you are consuming.

- Check the Percent Daily Values for nutritional guidelines.

- Check ingredients. Ingredients are listed in descending order by weight. Avoid products which list hydrogenated vegetable oils, coconut oil, or palm oil as one of the main ingredients.

Plain Rice

2	cups water
1	cup white or jasmine rice
¼	teaspoon salt

◉ In a medium saucepan, bring water, rice, and salt to a boil. Cover, reduce heat, and simmer about 20 minutes, until water is absorbed.

◉ Remove from heat, uncover, and let stand 5 minutes. Fluff rice with a fork.

Variations
Herbed Rice: Substitute chicken or vegetable broth for the water. When fluffing rice, stir in 2 tablespoons chopped fresh or 2 teaspoons dried basil, rosemary, or thyme.
Curried Rice: Substitute chicken broth for the water and add ½ teaspoon curry powder, ¼ teaspoon turmeric, and ½ cup raisins along with the salt.
Saffron Rice: Substitute chicken or vegetable broth for the water and add ⅛ teaspoon saffron along with the salt.

Makes 4 servings

Rice Pilaf

1	tablespoon butter/canola oil blend
1	teaspoon canola oil
½	cup diced onion (about 1 small onion)
½	cup diced celery (about 1 rib)
1	cup basmati rice
1	14½-oz. can chicken broth
½	cup dried fruit (e.g., raisins, cranberries, or chopped apricots)
½	teaspoon ground turmeric
⅛	teaspoon cinnamon
⅛	teaspoon black pepper

◉ In a medium saucepan heat butter and oil over medium heat. Add onion and celery and cook about 5 minutes. Stir in rice and cook 2 minutes.

◉ Add chicken broth, dried fruit, turmeric, cinnamon, and pepper and bring to a boil. Reduce heat, cover, and simmer about 20 minutes, until broth is absorbed.

◉ Remove from heat, uncover, and let stand 5 minutes. Fluff rice with a fork.

Makes 4 servings

Easy Spanish Rice

2	tablespoons olive oil
2	cups jasmine rice
1	14½-oz. can chicken broth
1	14½-oz. can diced tomatoes
1	4-oz. can diced green chili peppers, drained
1	cup diced onion (1 medium onion)
1	teaspoon minced garlic (about 2 medium cloves)
½	teaspoon salt
¼	teaspoon black pepper
¼	teaspoon cumin
	Pinch of saffron or ¼ teaspoon turmeric
1	cup frozen peas

◉ Heat olive oil in a deep skillet or Dutch oven over medium heat. Add rice and cook, stirring frequently, until rice is golden, about 5 minutes.

◉ Add broth, tomatoes, chili peppers, onion, garlic, salt, pepper, cumin, and saffron and bring to a boil. Cover, reduce heat, and simmer about 15 minutes, until most of the liquid is absorbed.

◉ Add peas, cover, and simmer another 5 minutes, until all the liquid is absorbed. Let stand 5 minutes before serving.

Makes 6–8 servings

Fried Rice

1	tablespoon canola oil
½	cup diced carrot (about 1 medium carrot)
½	cup diced onion (about 1 small onion)
3	cups cold, cooked white or jasmine rice
1	large egg, slightly beaten
1	tablespoon lite soy sauce
½	cup frozen peas, thawed

◉ Heat oil in skillet over medium-high heat. Add carrot and onion and cook, stirring frequently, about 7–10 minutes, until carrot is almost tender.

◉ Add rice and cook 3–5 minutes, stirring well, until heated through.

◉ Push rice to sides of skillet to make a well in the center. Add egg to center of skillet and cook, stirring well, about 2–3 minutes. Stir egg into rice. Add soy sauce and peas and cook 2–3 minutes more, until peas are heated through.

Makes 4 servings

Smoky Black Beans and Rice

This side dish will spice up a grilled chicken breast or roasted pork loin.

1½	tablespoons canola or olive oil
1	cup diced onion (about 1 medium onion)
½	cup diced red bell pepper (about ½ medium pepper)
½	teaspoon minced garlic (about 1 medium clove)
½	teaspoon cumin
¼	teaspoon coriander
¼	teaspoon salt
1	cup white rice
1	14½-oz. can chicken broth
1	15-oz. can black beans, rinsed and drained
	Reduced-fat sour cream (optional garnish)
	Plain yogurt (optional garnish)
	Chopped green onions (optional garnish)

◉ Heat canola oil in skillet over medium-high heat. Add onion and bell pepper and cook about 5 minutes. Add garlic and cook 1 minute more.

◉ Add cumin, coriander, salt, rice, and broth and bring to a boil. Cover, reduce heat, and simmer about 15 minutes, until most of the broth is absorbed.

◉ Stir in beans, cover, and simmer 5 minutes, until all broth has been absorbed.

◉ Garnish with sour cream, yogurt, and/or green onions, if desired.

Makes 6 servings

Cocktail Sauce

Depending on how hot you like your cocktail sauce, start with 1 tablespoon of horseradish, taste, and add more if you wish.

1	cup ketchup
1–2	tablespoons prepared horseradish
1	teaspoon Worcestershire sauce
1	teaspoon fresh lemon juice

◉ Combine all ingredients in a small bowl and mix well. Serve immediately or cover and chill.

Makes about 1 cup

Tartar Sauce

¾	cup Miracle Whip
¼	cup dill pickle relish
2	teaspoons fresh lemon juice
½	teaspoon prepared mustard

◉ Combine all ingredients in a small bowl and mix well. Serve immediately or cover and chill.

Makes about 1 cup

Horseradish Sauce

This sauce can be served with beef, pork, chicken, and fish. It can also be used as a sandwich spread. Opt for the yogurt if you are lactose intolerant.

½	cup Miracle Whip
½	cup lite sour cream or plain yogurt
3	tablespoons prepared horseradish

◉ Combine all ingredients in a small bowl and mix well. Serve immediately or cover and chill.

Makes about 1¼ cups

Barbecue Sauce

1	cup ketchup
½	cup dark brown sugar
2	tablespoons Worcestershire sauce
1½	tablespoons prepared mustard (yellow or Dijon)
1	tablespoon molasses
½	teaspoon salt
½	teaspoon onion powder
¼	teaspoon black pepper
2	dashes hot sauce, such as Texas Pete or Tabasco (optional)

◉ Combine all ingredients in a small saucepan and bring to a boil. Stir and boil 2 minutes. Use to baste meats or as a dipping sauce.

Makes about 1½ cups

Roasted Red Pepper Dipping Sauce

This lightly spiced dipping sauce compliments seafood and poultry. The long list of ingredients may seem daunting, but it comes together in minutes.

1	14-oz. jar roasted red peppers, drained
2	tablespoons cider vinegar
2	tablespoons tomato paste
2	tablespoons brown sugar
1	tablespoon olive or canola oil
$\frac{1}{2}$	teaspoon salt
$\frac{1}{4}$	teaspoon onion powder
$\frac{1}{4}$	teaspoon garlic powder
$\frac{1}{4}$	teaspoon paprika
$\frac{1}{8}$	teaspoon black pepper
$\frac{1}{8}$	teaspoon cumin
$\frac{1}{8}$	coriander
$\frac{1}{8}$	teaspoon cayenne (optional)

◉ Combine all ingredients in a food processor or blender and blend until smooth. Serve immediately or cover and chill.

Makes about 1 cup

Mango Chutney

Serve this chutney alongside a roasted pork loin or grilled chicken breast.

3	firm mangoes, peeled and chopped
½	cup brown sugar
½	cup raisins or dried cranberries
½	cup cider vinegar
1	cup diced onion (about 1 medium onion)
2	teaspoons fresh ginger, peeled and grated
1	teaspoon lemon zest (grated rind)
½	teaspoon cinnamon
¼	teaspoon cardamom

◉ Combine all ingredients in a large saucepan and bring to a boil. Reduce heat and simmer about 20 minutes, stirring occasionally. Cool, cover, and chill at least 2 hours before serving.

Variation
Peach Chutney: Substitute 5–6 medium peaches, peeled and chopped, for the mangos. Omit cardamom and add ⅛ teaspoon ground nutmeg.

Makes about 2 cups

Cranberry Sauce—Three Ways

Cranberry-Orange Sauce

1	12-oz. bag cranberries
¾	cup sugar
¼	cup brown sugar
½	cup orange juice
2	teaspoons orange zest (grated rind)
¼	teaspoon cinnamon
⅛	teaspoon ground ginger

Cranberry-Ginger Sauce

1	12-oz. bag cranberries
½	cup golden raisins
½	cup orange juice
½	cup brown sugar
2	tablespoons fresh ginger, peeled and grated
¼	teaspoon cinnamon
¼	teaspoon ground nutmeg

Cranberry-Horseradish Sauce

1	12-oz. bag cranberries
1	cup diced onion (about 1 medium onion)
¾	cup sugar
½	cup orange juice
3	tablespoons prepared horseradish

◉ Combine ingredients from recipe of choice above in a large saucepan and bring to a boil. Reduce heat and simmer about 10 minutes, stirring occasionally, until cranberries pop. Cool, cover, and chill at least 2 hours before serving.

Makes about 2 cups

Beet Relish

1	pound fresh beets, greens removed*
½	cup white vinegar
½	cup sugar
1	medium onion, cut in half and sliced thin
1	tablespoon prepared horseradish

◉ Place beets in a medium saucepan, cover with cold water, and bring to a boil. Reduce heat, cover, and simmer about 30 minutes, until tender—time will vary according to size of beets. Drain. When beets are cool enough to handle, peel and dice them.

◉ Combine vinegar and sugar in a medium saucepan and bring to a boil. Add onion, reduce heat, and simmer 5 minutes. Add beets and simmer 5 minutes. Remove from heat and stir in horseradish. Cool, cover, and chill at least 24 hours.

Note: For a shortcut, substitute canned beets for the fresh beets.

Makes about 2 cups

Sweet and Sour Pepper Relish

2	cups diced red bell peppers (about 2 medium peppers)
2	cups diced green bell peppers (about 2 medium peppers)
1	cup diced onion (about 1 medium onion)
1	cup white vinegar
¾	cup sugar
1	teaspoon salt
1	teaspoon mustard seeds

◉ Combine red and green peppers and onion in a Dutch oven, cover with cold water, and bring to a boil. Boil 5 minutes and then drain.

◉ Return vegetables to Dutch oven and add remaining ingredients. Bring to a boil and boil 5 minutes, stirring occasionally. Cool, cover, and chill 24 hours.

◉ Relish will keep about 1 month in refrigerator.

Makes about 2 pints

Standard Pastry Dough

TWO-CRUST PIE

2   cups all-purpose flour, plus more for dusting

1   teaspoon salt

⅔   cup vegetable shortening*

4–6   tablespoons cold water

◉ Combine flour and salt in a mixing bowl. Cut shortening into flour mixture with a pastry cutter or fork until crumbly. Add water, a little at a time, until dough is moist enough to almost form a ball—do not overmix as this will make the crust tough.

◉ Divide dough in half and shape into balls. On a floured surface, flatten dough into a disk. With a floured rolling pin, roll dough about 2 inches larger than your pie plate.

◉ Fold dough into quarters and place into pie plate. Unfold and press into bottom and sides of plate. Trim overhanging edges. Add desired filling.

◉ Roll second crust and fold into quarters. Cut 1-inch slits so steam can escape. Place on top of filling and unfold. Fold edges of top crust under edges of bottom crust and pinch to seal.

*Crisco brand now offers a vegetable shortening with no trans fats that has 50 percent less saturated fat than butter.

For a 1-Crust Pie: Cut ingredients in half. Trim overhanging edge and crimp edges.

Graham Cracker Crust

9	rectangular graham crackers, crushed (about 1½ cups)
2	tablespoons sugar
3	tablespoons butter/canola oil blend, melted

◉ Preheat oven to 350°F. Place crushed graham crackers in a 9-inch pie plate and sprinkle with sugar. Drizzle with melted butter and mix with fingers or fork until crumbs are evenly moistened.

◉ Press into bottom and sides of pie plate. Bake for 10 minutes and cool before filling.

Makes 1 crust

Bren's Apple Pie

The best apple pies are made from a combination of two different types of apples. Experiment with Cortland, Gala, Granny Smith, Jonathan, McIntosh, and Rome Beauty.

1	recipe 2-crust Standard Pastry Dough (pg. 197)
3	pounds apples (about 9 medium apples), peeled, cored, and sliced
½	cup sugar
¼	cup dark brown sugar
¼	cup all-purpose flour
½	teaspoon cinnamon
¼	teaspoon ground nutmeg
⅛	teaspoon salt
1	tablespoon butter/canola oil blend

◉ Preheat oven to 425°F. Line pie plate with rolled pastry dough.

◉ In a large bowl combine apple slices, sugar, brown sugar, flour, cinnamon, nutmeg, and salt; toss well to coat. Spoon into pastry-lined pie plate. Dot with butter broken into 3 or 4 pieces.

◉ Cover with second rolled pastry dough; fold edges and crimp. Cover edge of pie loosely with foil. Cover a baking sheet with foil to catch any overflow of juices. Place pie on baking sheet. Bake 30 minutes.

◉ Remove foil from pie and bake 20–25 minutes more, until crust is golden and juices begin to bubble through slits.

Variations
Apple-Cranberry Pie: Substitute 1 cup fresh cranberries for 1 of the apples.
Peach Pie: Substitute peeled, pitted, and sliced peaches (about 9 large) for the apples.

Makes 8–10 servings

Fresh Blueberry Pie

1	recipe 2-crust Standard Pastry Dough (pg. 197)
3	pints blueberries
½	cup sugar
½	cup all-purpose flour
½	teaspoon cinnamon
⅛	teaspoon salt
1	tablespoon butter/canola oil blend

◉ Preheat oven to 425°F. Line pie plate with rolled pastry dough.

◉ In a large bowl combine blueberries, sugar, flour, cinnamon, and salt; toss to coat. Spoon into pastry-lined pie plate. Dot with butter broken into 3 or 4 pieces.

◉ Cover with second rolled pastry dough; fold edges and crimp. Cover edge of pie loosely with foil. Cover a baking sheet with foil to catch any overflow of juices. Place pie on baking sheet. Bake 30 minutes.

◉ Remove foil from pie and bake 15–20 minutes more, until crust is golden and juices begin to bubble through slits.

Makes 8–10 servings

Cherry Pie

1	recipe 2-crust Standard Pastry Dough (pg. 197)
2	16-oz. cans pitted tart cherries, drained
1	cup sugar
½	cup all-purpose flour
½	teaspoon almond or vanilla extract
1	tablespoon butter/canola oil blend

◉ Preheat oven to 425°F. Line pie plate with rolled pastry dough.

◉ In a bowl combine cherries, sugar, flour, and almond extract; toss to coat. Spoon into pastry-lined pie plate. Dot with butter broken into 3 or 4 pieces.

◉ Cover with second rolled pastry dough; fold edges and crimp. Cover edge of pie loosely with foil. Cover a baking sheet with foil to catch any overflow of juices. Place pie on baking sheet. Bake 30 minutes.

◉ Remove foil from pie and bake 15–20 minutes more, until crust is golden and juices begin to bubble through slits.

Makes 8–10 servings

Strawberry Rhubarb Pie

1	recipe 2-crust Standard Pastry Dough (pg. 197)
3	cups fresh rhubarb, cut in ½-inch slices (about 1 pound)
4	cups strawberries, stemmed and sliced (about 1 quart)
1¼	cups sugar
½	cup flour
1	tablespoon butter/canola oil blend

- Preheat oven to 425°F. Line pie plate with rolled pastry dough.

- In a large bowl combine rhubarb, strawberries, sugar, and flour; toss well to coat. Spoon into pastry-lined pie plate. Dot with butter broken into 3 or 4 pieces.

- Cover with second rolled pastry dough; fold edges and crimp. Cover edge of pie loosely with foil. Cover a baking sheet with foil to catch any overflow of juices. Place pie on baking sheet. Bake 30 minutes.

- Remove foil from pie and bake 20–25 minutes more, until crust is golden and juices begin to bubble through slits.

Makes 8–10 servings

Pumpkin Pie

Pumpkin pie is a tasty way to incorporate more fiber in your diet. You needn't serve it only at Thanksgiving or Christmas—enjoy it anytime.

1	recipe 1-crust Standard Pastry Dough (pg. 197)
2	large eggs, slightly beaten
1	15-oz. can solid-pack pumpkin
1	12-oz. can fat-free evaporated milk or 1½ cups soy milk
½	cup sugar
¼	cup dark brown sugar
1	teaspoon cinnamon
½	teaspoon salt
½	teaspoon ground ginger
¼	teaspoon ground nutmeg
⅛	teaspoon ground cloves

◉ Preheat oven to 425°F. Line pie plate with rolled pastry dough and crimp edges. Place prepared pie plate on a foil-lined baking sheet.

◉ Place remaining ingredients in a mixing bowl and whisk thoroughly to combine. Pour into pastry shell. Cover edge of pie loosely with foil. Bake 15 minutes. Reduce oven temperature to 375°F and bake 30 minutes.

◉ Remove foil from pie and bake 20–25 minutes more, until knife inserted in center comes out clean.

Makes 8 servings

Key Lime Pie

If fresh key limes are available, by all means, use them. This recipe is lower in fat than traditional key lime pie, but it is not low in lactose.

1	14-oz. can fat-free sweetened condensed milk
2	large eggs, slightly beaten
½	cup bottled key lime juice
2	teaspoons lime zest (grated rind)
1	recipe Graham Cracker Crust (pg. 198)
1	lime, thinly sliced (optional)

◉ Preheat oven to 350°F. Whisk together sweetened condensed milk, eggs, lime juice, and lime zest until combined and thickened. Pour into prepared crust and bake 20 minutes. Cool completely. Chill for at least 2 hours before serving. Garnish with slices of lime, if desired.

Makes 8 servings

Strawberry Cheesecake Pie

This recipe is not for those who are lactose intolerant.

2	8-oz. packages reduced-fat cream cheese, softened
½	cup sugar
1	teaspoon vanilla extract
2	large eggs
1	recipe Graham Cracker Crust (pg. 198)
2	cups strawberries, stemmed and cut in half from top to tip (about 1 pint
½	cup seedless strawberry jam

◉ Preheat oven to 350°F. Beat cream cheese, sugar, and vanilla in a mixing bowl until fluffy. Beat in eggs, one at a time, until thoroughly combined.

◉ Pour into prepared crust and bake 25–30 minutes, until center is set. Cool completely. Arrange strawberry halves, cut side down, on top of cheesecake. Heat jam until melted and drizzle over strawberries.

◉ Chill 2–3 hours before serving.

Variations

Any number of toppings may be substituted for the strawberries and strawberry jam. Whole raspberries and seedless raspberry jam, whole blueberries and apricot jam, or pitted tart cherries and cherry jam are a few suggestions.

Makes 8–10 servings

Apples and Spice Crisp

5	cups peeled, cored, and sliced apples (about 5 medium apples)*
½	cup brown sugar
½	cup old-fashioned or quick oats
½	cup all-purpose flour
½	teaspoon cinnamon
¼	teaspoon ground nutmeg
4	tablespoons butter/canola oil blend, softened

◉ Preheat oven to 375°F. Coat a 2-quart casserole or an 8-inch square baking dish with vegetable spray. Arrange apple slices in the prepared dish.

◉ In a bowl combine brown sugar, oats, flour, cinnamon, nutmeg, and butter and mix well. Sprinkle over apples.

◉ Bake 30–35 minutes, until top is golden and apples are tender. Best when served warm.

Try pairing 2 varieties of apples for even more flavor such as: Cortland and Galas, Galas and McIntosh, McIntosh and Granny Smith, Granny Smith and Rome Beauty, or Rome Beauty and Cortland. Lots of possibilities!

Variations
Apple Cranberry Crisp: Substitute 2 cups cranberries tossed with ½ cup sugar for 2 cups of the apples.
Blueberry Crisp: Substitute 2 pints blueberries for the apples and omit nutmeg.
Peach Crisp: Substitute peeled, pitted, and sliced peaches (about 5 large) for the apples.

Makes 6 servings

Angel Food Cupcakes

6	large egg whites, room temperature
¾	teaspoon cream of tartar
⅛	teaspoon salt
½	cup sugar
½	teaspoon vanilla extract
¼	teaspoon almond extract
½	cup all-purpose flour, sifted

◉ Preheat oven to 375°F. With hand mixer, beat egg whites, cream of tartar, and salt in a mixing bowl until soft peaks form (when beaters are lifted). Add sugar, 2 tablespoons at a time, and beat until stiff peaks form. With a spatula, fold in vanilla and almond extracts. Sprinkle with flour, ¼ cup at a time, and fold in.

◉ Line a muffin pan with paper baking cups. Fill cups two-thirds full. Bake about 10–12 minutes, until golden and cake springs back when touched. Remove from pan and cool on wire rack. Serve with Sweet Berries (recipe below), if desired.

Variation
Chocolate Angel Food Cupcakes: Substitute 2 tablespoons cocoa for 2 tablespoons of the flour and resift. Omit almond extract.

Makes 12–15 cupcakes

Sweet Berries

2	cups fresh strawberries, stems removed and cut in half (about 1 pint)
1½	tablespoons sugar

◉ Place 1 cup of the strawberries in a bowl and mash. Add remaining berries, sprinkle with sugar, and toss to coat. Cover and chill 1 hour before serving.

Makes 2 cups

Gingerbread

⅓   cup applesauce

3   tablespoons butter/canola oil blend

½   cup brown sugar

1   large egg

1   cup molasses

½   cup hot water

2   cups all-purpose flour

1   teaspoon baking soda

1   teaspoon ground ginger

1   teaspoon cinnamon

½   teaspoon salt

¼   teaspoon ground nutmeg

     Powdered sugar (optional)

◉ Preheat oven to 350°F. Coat a 9-inch square baking dish with vegetable spray and lightly dust with flour.

◉ Place all ingredients except powdered sugar in a large bowl and beat with a hand mixer to combine. Beat another 2 minutes on medium speed. Pour batter into prepared dish and bake 35–45 minutes, until toothpick inserted in center comes out clean.

◉ Sprinkle with powdered sugar, if desired, or serve with Lemon Sauce (pg. 209) or Maple Sauce (pg. 209).

Makes 9 servings

Lemon Sauce

¾   cup water

½   cup sugar

1   tablespoon cornstarch

¼   cup fresh lemon juice (about 1½ lemons)

1   tablespoon lemon zest (grated rind)

      Pinch of ground nutmeg

      Pinch of salt

1   tablespoon butter/canola oil blend

◉ Bring water to a boil in a small saucepan. Add sugar and cornstarch and boil 1 minute, stirring constantly. Add lemon juice, lemon zest, nutmeg, and salt and bring back to a boil. Boil, stirring constantly, until smooth and thickened, about 5 minutes. Remove from heat and stir in butter. Serve warm.

Makes about 1 cup

Maple Sauce

½   cup pure maple syrup

½   cup brown sugar

¼   teaspoon salt

1   tablespoon butter/canola oil blend

½   teaspoon vanilla extract

◉ Combine maple syrup, brown sugar, and salt in a small saucepan over low-medium heat and bring to a boil. Boil about 5 minutes, stirring constantly, until thickened. Remove from heat and stir in butter and vanilla. Serve warm.

Makes about ½ cup

Peach Upside-Down Cake

4	cups peeled, pitted, and sliced peaches (about 4 large peaches)
¼	cup brown sugar
2	tablespoons butter/canola oil blend, melted
¼	cup butter/canola oil blend, softened
⅔	cup sugar
1	large egg
1	teaspoon vanilla extract
⅓	cup buttermilk or soy milk
1¼	cups all-purpose flour
1	teaspoon baking powder
½	teaspoon salt
¼	teaspoon cinnamon
⅛	teaspoon ground nutmeg

◉ Preheat oven to 350°F. Coat a 9-inch square baking dish with vegetable spray.

◉ Combine peaches, brown sugar, and 2 tablespoons melted butter in a bowl and toss to coat. Spoon into prepared dish.

◉ Cream together ¼ cup softened butter with sugar in a mixing bowl with a hand mixer. Add egg, vanilla, and buttermilk and mix well.

◉ Add flour, baking powder, salt, cinnamon, and nutmeg and mix well. Pour batter on top of peaches. Bake 35–45 minutes, until toothpick inserted in center comes out clean. Cool about 10–15 minutes. Serve warm.

Makes 9 servings

Oatmeal Cookies

½	cup butter/canola oil, softened
½	cup sugar
½	cup dark brown sugar
1	large egg
1½	teaspoons vanilla extract
¾	cup all-purpose flour
½	teaspoon baking soda
½	teaspoon salt
½	teaspoon cinnamon
¼	teaspoon ground nutmeg
1½	cups quick or old-fashioned oats
½	cup raisins (optional)

◉ Preheat oven to 350°F. Cream together softened butter, sugar, and brown sugar in a mixing bowl with a hand mixer. Beat in egg and vanilla.

◉ Add flour, baking soda, salt, cinnamon, and nutmeg and beat to combine. Stir in oats and raisins, if desired.

◉ Drop dough by heaping teaspoonfuls about 2 inches apart onto an ungreased baking sheet. Bake 10 minutes for a chewy cookie or 12 minutes for a crispy cookie. Cool on wire rack.

Makes about 2½ dozen cookies

Peanut Butter Cookies

You can substitute almond, cashew, or soy nut butter for the peanut butter in this recipe if you wish—they are all delicious.

1	cup natural creamy-style peanut butter (no hydrogenated oils)
½	cup butter/canola oil blend, softened
½	cup sugar plus 1–2 teaspoons more to shape cookies
½	cup dark brown sugar
1	large egg
1¼	cups all-purpose flour
½	teaspoon baking powder
½	teaspoon baking soda
¼	teaspoon salt

◉ Preheat oven to 375°F. Cream together peanut butter, butter, ½ cup sugar, brown sugar, and egg in a mixing bowl with a hand mixer.

◉ Add the flour, baking powder, baking soda, and salt and beat to combine. Shape dough into 1-inch balls and place 2 inches apart on an ungreased baking sheet. Using a fork dipped in sugar, flatten cookies with a crisscross pattern. Bake 8–10 minutes until set. Cool on wire rack.

Makes about 3 dozen cookies

Molasses Cookies

½   cup sugar plus 1–2 tablespoons more for rolling cookies

½   cup brown sugar

¾   cup vegetable shortening*

¼   cup molasses

1   large egg

2   cups all-purpose flour

2   teaspoons baking soda

1   teaspoon cinnamon

1   teaspoon ground ginger

¼   teaspoon ground nutmeg

¼   teaspoon salt

◉ Preheat oven to 375°F. Cream together ½ cup sugar, brown sugar, shortening, molasses, and egg in a mixing bowl with a hand mixer.

◉ Add the flour, baking soda, cinnamon, ginger, nutmeg, and salt and beat to combine. Shape dough into 1-inch balls, roll in sugar, and place about 3 inches apart on an un-greased baking sheet. Bake about 10 minutes, until set. Cool on wire rack.

Crisco brand now offers a vegetable shortening with no trans fats—look for the green label.

Makes about 3 dozen cookies

Ginger Cookies

½	cup butter/canola oil blend, softened
½	cup molasses
½	cup dark brown sugar
1	large egg
2½	cups all-purpose flour
1½	teaspoons ground ginger
1	teaspoon baking soda
½	teaspoon salt
½	teaspoon cinnamon
¼	teaspoon ground cloves
⅛	teaspoon ground nutmeg
1–2	tablespoons sugar

- Preheat oven to 375°F. Cream together butter, molasses, and brown sugar in a mixing bowl with a hand mixer. Add egg and beat to combine.

- Add flour, ginger, baking soda, salt, cinnamon, cloves, and nutmeg and beat to combine.

- Shape dough into 1½-inch balls, roll in sugar, and place 2 inches apart on an ungreased baking sheet. Bake about 10 minutes until set. Cool cookies 1 minute on the baking sheet then transfer to wire rack to cool completely.

Makes about 3 dozen cookies

Lemon Ice Box Cookies

The dough for these old-fashioned cookies can be made ahead and kept on hand in the refrigerator for up to a week or frozen* for up to 1 month in a ziplock freezer bag.

½	cup butter/canola oil blend, softened
1	cup sugar
1	large egg
2	tablespoons fresh lemon juice (about 1 small lemon)
2	teaspoons lemon zest (grated rind)
2	cups all-purpose flour
1	teaspoon baking powder
¼	teaspoon baking soda
¼	teaspoon salt

◉ Cream together butter and sugar in a mixing bowl with a hand mixer. Add egg, lemon juice, and lemon zest and beat to combine.

◉ Add flour, baking powder, baking soda, and salt and beat to combine. Divide dough in half and shape into 12-inch logs on waxed paper. Wrap logs up in waxed paper and chill overnight (at least 8 hours).

◉ Preheat oven to 375°F. Cut logs into ½-inch slices and place 2 inches apart on an ungreased baking sheet. Bake about 12–14 minutes, until edges are golden. Cool on wire rack.

Note: If using frozen dough, thaw overnight in the refrigerator before baking.

Makes about 3½ dozen cookies

Jam-Filled Oatmeal Bars

½	cup butter/canola oil blend, softened
½	cup sugar
½	cup brown sugar
1	large egg
1	cup all-purpose flour
½	teaspoon cinnamon
¼	teaspoon salt
1	cup quick or old-fashioned oats
1	cup seedless strawberry or raspberry jam

◉ Preheat oven to 350°F. Coat a 9-inch square baking dish with vegetable spray.

◉ In a mixing bowl cream the butter, sugar, and brown sugar with hand mixer. Add egg and beat to combine. Add flour, cinnamon, and salt and beat to combine. Stir in oats.

◉ Press half of crumb mixture into prepared pan. Spread with jam and sprinkle remaining crumb mixture on top. Bake 35–40 minutes until golden. Cool completely before cutting into bars.

Makes 16 bars

Cocoa Brownies

Try these with a scoop of vanilla frozen yogurt and Sweet Berries (pg. 207).

½ cup butter/canola oil blend, melted

1 cup sugar

2 large eggs

1½ teaspoons vanilla extract

½ cup unsweetened cocoa or carob powder

½ cup all-purpose flour

1 teaspoon baking powder

½ teaspoon salt

◉ Preheat oven to 350°F. Coat an 8-inch square baking dish with vegetable spray.

◉ In a mixing bowl combine melted butter, sugar, eggs, and vanilla and stir until well mixed. Stir in the cocoa, flour, baking powder, and salt just until combined.

◉ Spread batter in prepared baking dish and bake 25–30 minutes, until toothpick inserted in center comes out clean. Cool completely before cutting into bars.

Variation
Blondies: Omit cocoa or carob powder. Substitute brown sugar for the granulated sugar.

Makes 16 brownies

Suggested Further Reading

American Heart Association and American Cancer Society. *Living Well, Staying Well: Big Health Rewards from Small Lifestyle Changes.* New York: Times Books, 1996.

Balch, Phyllis A., CNC. *Prescription for Nutritional Healing: The A-Z Guide to Supplements.* 2nd ed. New York: Avery, 2002.

Bonci, Leslie, MPH, RD. *American Dietetic Association Guide to Better Digestion.* New York: John Wiley and Sons, Inc., 2003.

Foods That Harm Foods That Heal: An A-Z Guide to Safe and Healthy Eating. Pleasantville, NY: Reader's Digest, 1997.

Hoffmann, David, BSc, FNIMH. *Healthy Digestion: A Natural Approach to Relieving Indigestion, Gas, Heartburn, Constipation, Colitis, and More.* Pownal, VT: Storey Books, 2000.

Mount Sinai School of Medicine. *Total Nutrition: The Only Guide You'll Ever Need.* Edited by Victor Herbert and Genell J. Subak-Sharpe. New York: St. Martin's Press, 1995.

Murray, Michael, ND, and Joseph Pizzorno, ND. *Encyclopedia of Natural Medicine.* Rocklin, CA: Prima Publishing, 1998.

Saibil, Fred, MD. *Crohn's Disease and Ulcerative Colitis: Everything You Need to Know.* Buffalo, NY: Firefly Books, 2003.

Wills, Judith. *The Food Bible.* A Fireside book. New York: Simon and Schuster, 1998.

Winter, Ruth, MS. *A Consumer's Dictionary of Food Additives.* New York: Three Rivers Press, 1999.

Yoshida, Cynthia M., MD. *No More Digestive Problems.* New York: Bantam Dell, 2004.

Helpful Web Sites

Crohn's and Colitis Foundation of America
www.ccfa.org

www.mayoclinic.com

www.medlineplus.gov

www.nutrition.gov

www.webmd.com

Mount Sinai Medical Center
www.msmc.com

Johns Hopkins Medicine
www.hopkinsmedicine.org

www.sciencedaily.com

National Institutes of Health
www.nih.gov

Index